W9-AKA-056

# Lotions, Potions, and Deadly Elixirs

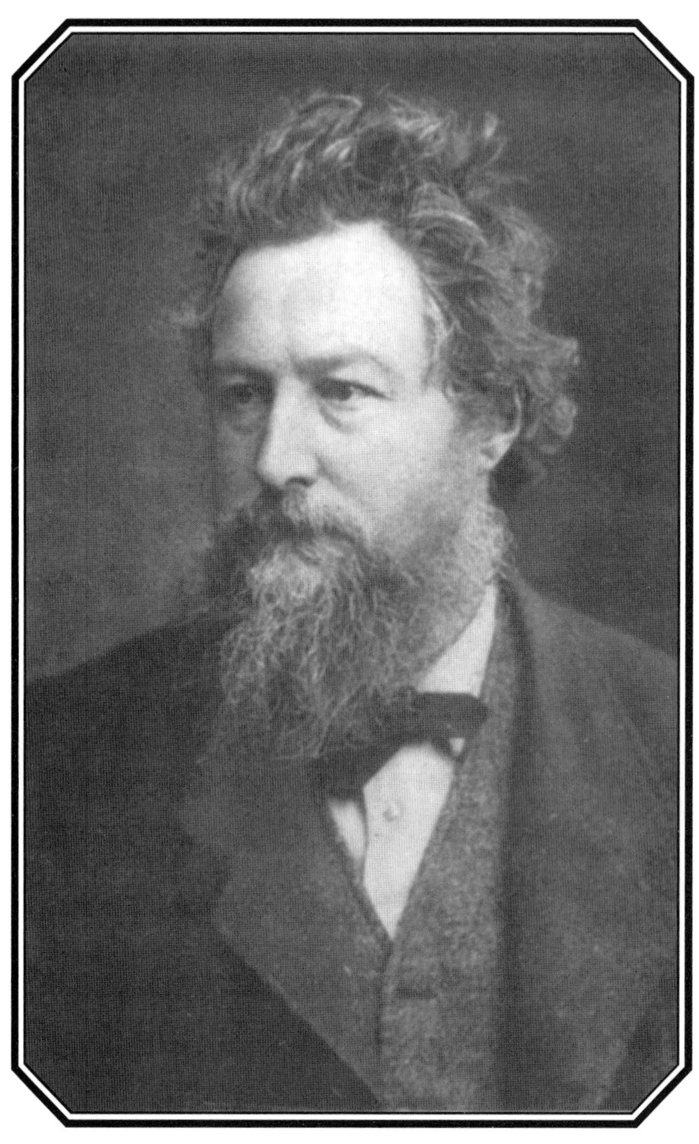

Yea, why then was I born, since hope is pain,
And life a lingering death, and faith but vain,
And love the loss of all I seemed to gain?
—ROBERT MORRIS, from *On the Edge of Wilderness*

# Lotions, Potions, and Deadly Elixirs

## *Frontier Medicine in America*

WAYNE BETHARD

A Roberts Rinehart Book
TAYLOR TRADE PUBLISHING
*Lanham New York Toronto Oxford*

Taylor Trade
A Roberts Rinehart Book
A wholly owned subsidiary of The Rowman & Littlefield Publishing Group, Inc.
4501 Forbes Boulevard, Suite 200
Lanham, MD 20706

Distributed by National Book Network

*Library of Congress Cataloging-in-Publication Data*

Bethard, Wayne.

Lotions, potions, and deadly elixirs : frontier medicine in America / Wayne Bethard.

p. cm.

Includes bibliographical references and index.

ISBN 1-57098-432-8 (hardcover : alk. paper)

1. Medicine—United States—History—18th century. 2. Medicine—United States—History—19th century. 3. Pharmacology—United States—History—18th century. 4. Pharmacology—United States—History—19th century. I. Title.

R151.B38 2004

610'.973—dc22 2003021820

∞ The paper used in this publication meets the minimum requirements of American National Standard for Information Sciences—Permanence of Paper for Printed Library Materials, ANSI/NISO Z39.48-1992.

*Manufactured in the United States of America.*

*To Leorah*

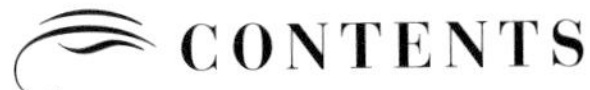

# CONTENTS

## Two Treatments: The Good, the Sad, and the Ungodly 29

# FOREWORD

A FEW NOVELS AGO, I decided to get rid of several minor characters. They'd served their purposes and were cluttering the story. The setting was the Texas Panhandle in 1873. I considered a Kiowa raid and buffalo stampede to get rid of them, but I opted instead for cholera, a biological equivalent of the Gatling gun. Too bad I didn't have a copy of Wayne Bethard's *Lotions, Potions, and Deadly Elixirs: Frontier Medicine in America*. My doomed characters might have suffered from dyspepsia, dropsy, and gravel, which could have been treated in vain with sulfur or calcic water. Raiders could have inflicted wounds later cauterized by a glowing poker daubed with pine tar and gunpowder. The path to perdition would have been smoothed by gum of raw opium or laudanum. In short, I could have told a better story.

I won't be caught lacking again. *Lotions, Potions, and Deadly Elixirs: Frontier Medicine in America* deserves a prominent place in the library of every historian, historical novelist, and anyone who enjoys a good story. Yes, Wayne Bethard is a registered pharmacist and exacting researcher. But he's also a novelist, veteran outdoor writer, and humorist who never takes himself too seriously.

In this book, you'll learn the truth about tars, paints, swabs, folding powders, and other dosage forms. The pioneer drug monographs will educate you as to the medicinal value of barbed wire and horseshoe nails, apple cider vinegar, arsenic, and madstones. You'll learn archaic terms for ailments and treatments (did one lance a furuncle or have a painful eructation?), and, most important, you'll be entertained by stories of a real Dr. Quinn, Medicine Woman, as well as Ben Franklin's turpentine pill and other examples of frontier medical heroism and quackery.

For years, Wayne has honed his craft writing for various outdoor magazines and entertaining the members of The DFW Writers' Workshop with his stories. His readers are the beneficiaries of patient and dedicated work. In this book he brings together his pharmaceutical expertise with his love of history and storytelling. As a western novelist, he recognized a need in the current reference material and filled it.

So have a seat at the drugstore soda fountain and relax while the good druggist prepares your nostrums and mixes your elixirs. You're in capable hands.

HENRY CHAPPELL

## ACKNOWLEDGMENTS

BETWEEN EVERY GOLDEN EGG, there is bound to be a little mass and gas. I would like to thank everyone who assisted me with this little egg, especially the DFW Writers Workshop, who helped me clean up my masses. A special thanks goes to Erin McKindley and her wonderful copy-editing staff, who waved their laced editing fans to whisk away the many pungent blunders that had escaped me. I also thank my wife for putting up with me during all this; my professors and the helpful staff at the University of Texas College of Pharmacy; John Lovett, assistant curator of the University of Oklahoma Western History Collection; Russell Stocks and Julie Henderson for their help with bezoars; Art Weaver for his mineral wells pictures; the Hughes Springs Chamber of Commerce; Susan Black, my research librarian at the Longview Public Library; and all the professors, physicians, and pharmacists who went out of their way to lend a hand.


### DISCLAIMER

This author has attempted to assemble a suitable information base on medicines used in America's frontier times. Mistakenness, errors, or blunders are always possible even in reputable reference materials. Neither the author nor the publisher assumes responsibility for inaccuracies or patient care associated with the applications of information contained in this presentation. People not of the health profession should seek appropriate professional supervi-

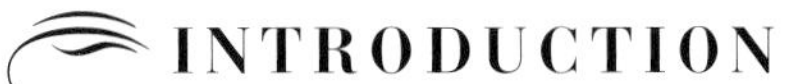

# INTRODUCTION

NO, WHEN I GREW UP I didn't walk barefoot in the snow, uphill both ways, ten miles to town, or carry my lunch to school in a lard bucket. I do remember the good old days though: Momma warming my sausage biscuits in her old kerosene microwave, her leaning over the kitchen sink cutting the curly tips off the spaghetti she grew in her window-box garden.

Seriously, I did carry my lunch to school in a can, but mine had an embossed picture of Roy Rogers on it. I wish I still had that old lunch box. I remember my mother treating my childhood ills, too. How can I forget that sticky Vicks salve washrag stuck to my chest? And those nasty-tasting, bitter-licorice liquids she poured down me. To this day, I can't drink orange juice without the taste of castor oil flagging a thought. Oh, yeah, I remember my first, and last, exposure to Dr. Caldwell's laxative, too. It was on a Saturday afternoon back in '63. I was sitting in the den with my two brothers and my dad. Texas was vying for a national football championship, as I recall, when Mother waltzed into the room with a tablespoon in one hand and a black bottle in the other. She purposely stood in our way until we each took a dose of that stinky stuff. It was the only way we could get rid of her. I'll never forget the next morning, either. Dad homesteaded the bathroom first. The rest of us just stood there in line, walking in place, fist clenched, knees together, as we listened to a lot of heavy breathing on the other side of the door.

I do believe, though, I felt better afterward, and the next day it didn't hurt me . . . unless I laughed.

Old farts who write about the past reminisce a lot. As you will see, I delight in reporting amusing historical facts but on numerous occasions, have been accused of dipping my quill in the well of thin manure.

People are all the time asking me questions about medicines. "Say, aren't you the expert on drugs?" My reply is usually, "Not unless, by 'expert,' you mean an old drip."

As that old country song goes, "I ain't no real cowboy, I just found this hat." I'm not a real cowboy. I don't ride the range and mend fences, but I am a real druggist, a certified, full-blooded, genuine, registered pharmacist, and the truest of all drugstore cowboys. A professional, I like to think.

The difference between a professor (a real expert) and a professional is that a professor knows it all. A professional simply knows where to look it all up, that or which professor to contact when he needs to know it all.

While attending pharmacy school at the University of Texas back in 1963, I had the occasion to study under some truly wonderful professors: Dr. C. C. Albers and Dr. Esther Jane Wood Hall. Dr. Hall was my counselor. I worked for her, grading exams; doing research and helping her write and edit some of her papers. She told me I had a natural way with words and that since I enjoyed writing so much, I should consider taking some writing courses as electives. I took the courses, and she was right—I loved it. While working under her, I helped with several projects, one of which was a piece on *Drugs Used on the Chisholm Trail.*

Recently, while doing research on the Internet for this book, I came across on a history Web site, specifically a piece on the history of Texas pharmacy. I read the first half of the article, skipped to the end, and smiled when I saw it was written by Esther Jane Wood Hall, my old professor. I downloaded the article, printed it, and handed it to my wife. "Here, read this," I said, smiling.

She took it and read.

When she neared the end of the article, I said, "Look who wrote it." She looked up with a straight face and said, "You did."

I hastily took the article back and read the last portion. With a straight face, I replied, "I'll be darned."

I really didn't write it all—Dr. Hall did most of it; I did help research and edit it, though. I will say this, that last part sure sounded good for some reason.

A lot of what appears in this book comes from a worn-out old memory. Where possible, I have backed up what I report with documented resources. Unfortunately, I don't have my old professors to call on anymore; they were all over sixty at the time I started pharmacy school.

Keep in mind as you read this book that historical medicine is a science based on facts compiled from research. Like anthropology or archeology, the history of any science is an evolving process. Every day new bones or remnants of dinosaurs are found, which totally change the facts as to when humans and animals were first thought to have come into being. Likewise, historical medical facts evolve, too. The dates listed in this book are based on my own research. If an old diary or documents are discovered that show these dates to be in error, if you're not a professor yourself, I'll proudly stand corrected, provided you send me a copy of the documentation. If you are a professor, don't beat me over the head with your knowledge; I might enjoy it.

Keep in mind, too, that many drugs underwent trial periods of a year or more before they proved their worth. Many dates listed in this book were the first dates the drugs appeared in official compendiums.

Medicines were more accessible in frontier times than one might suspect. Some drugs used then are still in use today. A few of these old medicines were pure poisons, some were just plain quackery, but many, as you will see, were quite effective, enjoyable-to-learn-about remedies. Sit back now and enjoy a trip down medical memory lane with the zany medicaments, predicaments, lotions, potions, and poisons that helped win our rugged west.

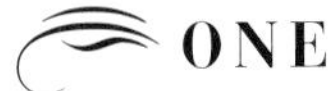 ONE

# *Frontier Dosage Forms*

MANY DOSAGE FORMS used on the frontier, like intimate moments caught in time, have been all but forgotten. To savor their uniqueness, this chapter enlightens as to how old drugs were prepared, packaged, and taken or given.

Frontier drugs came from all sources: plants, animals, and minerals. Those derived from plants were classed as herbs and vegetables, the ground-up or liquid extracts of leaves, roots, and barks; those from animals were prepared from kidneys, adrenal glands, and fats and skins, oils, and digestive ferments. Mineral medicaments came from inorganic salts and various chemicals, all of which were prepared in two forms, a dry form, and a liquid form.

The Wets were liquid forms of frontier medicines. Tonics were the bitters, aromatics, astringents, stimulants, and alteratives; any and all products, external or internal, were prepared in malleable or palatable fluid forms.

The Drys, like old cowboys, were ground up, desiccated, dried out, parched, and dehydrated—the waterless forms of medicines. That's not to say old cowboys were waterless, quite the contrary.

## THE WETS

### *The Mineral Acids*

Mineral acids were the inorganically derived liquids that aided general health by various means. Iron liquids were used to build blood. Elemental iron occurs in nature in two forms, the ferric and the ferrous form. The *ferric* is the form found in iron ore and water. It wasn't toxic when consumed, but it wasn't beneficial, either. An overabundance of ferric iron in the diet occurred mostly from consuming well water that had high concentrations of the mineral. Ferric iron was notorious for depositing in the teeth of growing children and leaving mottled, reddish, almost marblelike permanent stains on teeth.

*Ferrous iron* was the only iron form the body could use beneficially.

The mineral, phosphorus, found little use by itself but was thought to have a synergistic action with strychnine. Many old tonics were prepared in combination with nux vomica (frontier strychnine).

Mineral acids like nitric acid, muriatic acid, and sulphuric acid, in very small amounts, improved digestion. Refined muriatic, or hydrochloric, acid was the only acid of lasting medical value. Dilute solutions of hydrochloric acid were, and still are, used for achlorhydria (the absence of stomach acid). Nitric and sulfuric acids, save for manufacturing of other substances, found little use as medicines then or now. Sulfuric is the acid used in car batteries. Using battery acid to help digest a Big Mac doesn't sound appealing, does it? For sure, that's the kind of charge I can do without.

### *The Vegetable Acids*

Vegetable acids were organically derived and used to treat everything from headaches to sprains and bruises, as well as other acute skin ailments. Examples of vegetable acids are acetic acid, citric acid, and carbonic acid. Acetic acid is the acid in vinegar that preserves and pickles cucumbers, okra, and cabbage. Applying vinegar

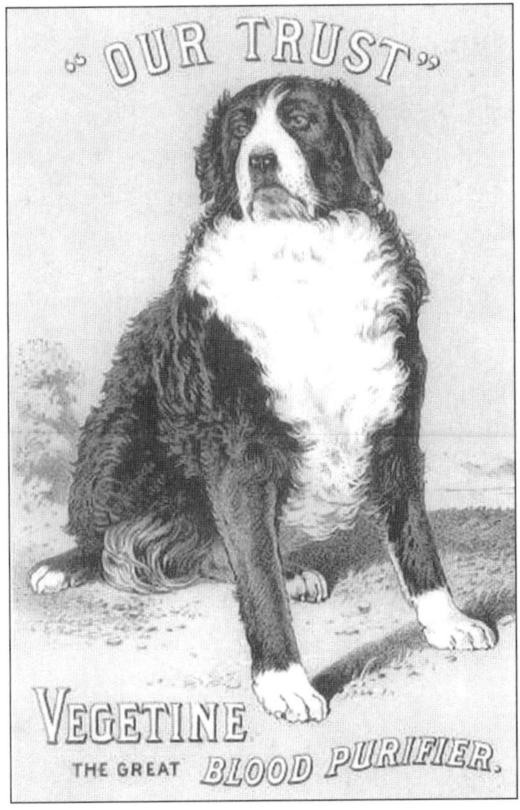


mildly pickled the top layers of the skin. Regardless of the smell, and the desire to bite oneself, vinegar helped relieve sunburn and similar skin irritations. When applied to irritated skin, vinegar makes skin sting before it feels better. That is perhaps why it found little favor in treating minor hemorrhoid flare-ups or burning bottoms caused from improper wipings with pine straw or leaves.

### *Tars, Paints, Swabs, and Other Disgusting Taints*

Monkeybloods and gentian violet were favorite forms of topical antiseptics. My other brother Don and I used to enjoy tattooing ourselves with them. The best of all was gentian violet. It stained the skin a dark, bluish purple, and, like Mercurochrome, it left a metallic sheen in its wake. I'll never forget the time my Aunt Willa Dean and Uncle Harold stayed with us all night once. Aunt Dean's nose was so stuffed up that every other word she spoke had a *w* in it. Sometime during the night, she reached for a jar of Vicks salve she'd brought with her and placed on the nightstand. In the darkness, and in the fogginess of her condition, she opened a similar-sized bottle of gentian violet Grandma kept on the same table to treat an ingrown toenail she had.

"Honey?" Aunt Dean said to her husband. "Is it hot in here to you?"

Uncle Harold grumbled and turned on the light. He woke up the whole house laughing. Aunt Dean had opened that bottle of gentian violet and swabbed her neck with it; she even ran some up her nose and licked her fingertips. She said she thought the Vicks salve was so thin because it was hot in the room and it had melted. Said she couldn't taste or smell nothing, so in the dark she ran some up her nose to help clear her nostrils.

Gentian violet on the skin is pert near-permanent. No one in our family wanted to be seen with Aunt Dean for a while. She looked like she'd been kicked in the throat by Grandpa's old mule, Kate. The look of shiny, purple snot running down her front lip didn't help.

I'll never forget that "gaggy" iodine the doctor swabbed our throats with, either. The smell of phenol still pinches a nerve in my mind when I whiff it. An iodine, phenol, and glycerin swabbing was the main treatment for strep throat back then. Boy, how I hated to see that long cotton-tipped swab coming at me. But at least being stained inside didn't look so bad. If you made it through the jerking from trying to keep down your lunch, it did help a sore throat.

Then there were the monkeybloods, Mercurochrome and Merthiolate, both of which colored the skin a bright metallic red. These were well-accepted treatments for cuts and sores. Bactine and Neosporin came much later.

Dab the wound with monkeyblood, cover it with a strip of cloth, and voilà, you got well. I always thought of how Grandma tore strips from an old pillowcase or sheet and tied the ends around our finger or hand. We used to gather around and watch when another kid unwrapped a bandage to expose that red badge of courage. Morbid amusement, I guess, but to this day, I still can't resist looking when someone removes a bandage to expose the pruney and white the skin around a wound.

Another paint that stains the skin was the antiseptic silver nitrate. It turned the skin black.

The tars—coal tar, pine tar, and creosotes—were most useful for their carbolic acid content. Volatile phenols were prepared by the destructive distillation of plants. Phenol-containing preparations like thyme, clove, pimenta, myrcia oil, rectified birch tar oil, creosote, pine tar, juniper tar, and coal tar were used for their topical disinfectant action and for deadening the pain of abscesses and other eruptive skin conditions like psoriasis and saddle sores. A dab of juniper tar at the end of a hard day's ride (after it finally quit burning) did wonders for a sore arse.

Coal tars compounded into moisturizing ointments and creams are still used to this day by dermatologists to treat psoriasis and other similar skin irritations. In the old days, the gummy grease was gathered from open tar pits, bottled and sold to treat practically everything topical.

Back when I was younger, country folks had a serious problem with screwworms that infected their cattle. Screwworms weren't like green fly maggots that ate dead flesh only; they ate live flesh and most of the time killed the cow. Why they called it being "blown" I'll never know, but I can't count the number of times I heard Gramps say that a cow's wound got blown by screwworms.

Aside from tinkling all the time, Gramps had psoriasis on his elbows—nasty lesions he never got totally rid of, but that got better when Grandma treated him with LeGear's Screw Worm Killer. That smell, along with the methyl-salicylate analgesic (the Ben-Gay) stench that suffocated you when you entered Gramps's bedroom, reminds me of him. When you look at the old Legear's formula, you see that it contained mostly coal tar.

Grandma used a lot of veterinary medicines on herself and us.

She applied udder balm to her heels at night, Absorbine veterinary liniment to her aching back and joints, and screwworm killer to Gramps's scaly elbows. By the way, she made a paste with gentian violet to dab on the "pecking" sores on her baby chickens. She simply did what most people did back then: used what she had.

Grandma Haley cooked her fried chicken in pure hog lard, ate real butter on her biscuits, fried and scarfed down six pieces of bacon or sausage every morning, along with the three or four eggs she fried in hog lard. And she dipped snuff, the bad kind—Garrett's Sweet, as I remember. Grandma lived to be ninety-four years old. Isn't there something wrong with this picture?

## *Astringents, Expectorants, Tinctures and Fluidextracts, Bitters, Blisters, Tonics, Waters, and Wines*

The word astringent comes from Latin and means "to draw or contract." Astringents work by locally stimulating the muscles in the outer layers of the skin. My most memorable experiences with astringents were back in junior high school. That was when pimples, or "zits," as we called them, were a plague to us macho handsome beings. I remember how tight that old acne lotion made my face feel, so tight it made my face shiny, and as big as my nose was back then, that was a lot of shine.

Blisters were corrosive agents that caused pain and made the skin whelp and blister. Ironically, they were used to treat pain. Frontiersmen didn't know how they worked; they just knew that they did. The old medical theory was based on *epispastos*, the Greek word meaning "to draw on oneself by attracting the humors of the skin," *humors* being the liquids in the body, the condition and proportions of which bodily health and mental health were supposed to depend. The real basis for their action was by causing the release of endorphins. Endorphins, the body's natural painkiller, gave the patient the equivalent of a runner's high and did indeed help relieve pain—the old, "make it hurt worse somewhere else."

A tincture is a solution of the active principles, chiefly vegetable, sometimes of saline medicinals or animal origin, dissolved in a solvent. There were several types of tinctures depending on their solvent: *alcoholic tinctures* use alcohol as a solvent. *Ethereal tinctures* use sulphuric ether as a solvent. *Ammoniated tinctures* use ammonia as a solvent. If wine is used as a solvent for a medicine, it isn't called a wine tincture; it's called a *medicinal wine.*

There were simple tinctures and compound tinctures. *Simple tinctures* contained only one active substance or drug in solution; *compound tinctures* contained two or more. The old Merthiolates and iodines were simple tinctures. Benzoin tincture was a compound tincture.

The majority of tinctures were prepared in alcohol. Those for internal use were prepared in ethanol (grain alcohol—the drinking kind). The most memorable of all oral tinctures was a standardized preparation containing the active ingredients of opium. Tincture of opium is still available and used today. Topical tinctures of iodine and Merthiolate were prepared in isopropyl or denatured alcohol and are no longer available.

A fluidextract is a liquid preparation of vegetable drugs that contain alcohol as preservative or solvent, or both, and whose volume is equal to a measure of distilled water, which weighs the same as the drug being dissolved—in other words, a 1:1 mixture. There are simple fluidextracts and compound fluidextracts. Most fluids extracts are prepared by percolation.

The word expectorant evolves from the Latin word *expectorate*, which means "to eject from the mouth by the hacking, coughing, or spitting up of mucous or phlegm or other discharge from the throat or lungs"—the old "fling a lugie," so to speak. An expectorant is any drug, chemical, food, or agent that thins or liquefies phlegm in the throat or chest and makes it easier to get rid of by coughing.

Bitters, a notorious form of frontier medicines, came as *simple bitters.* Of vegetable origin, they were used to improve appetite and expand digestive powers. Examples are barberry, boneset, dogwood,

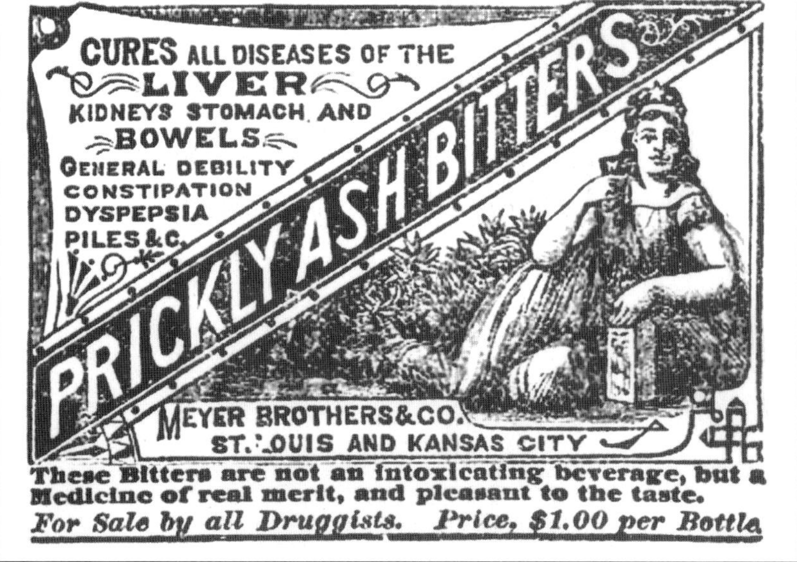


guassia, gentian, and columba. Another class of bitters were the *aromatic bitters*, which actively stimulated the digestive system: chamomile, Virginia snakeroot, cascarilla, angostura, cinnamon, clove, nutmeg, allspice, ginger, and various peppers (the active ingredient of which was capsicum).

Bitters were prepared by steeping herbs or roots in spirituous liquors. They got their name from the "sour" taste imparted by the active ingredients in the plants. The name became synonymous with any tonic, elixir, or alcohol-containing liquid, which was used to treat stomach ailments or, if they contained anodynes, pain. If it helped ease the gut or stop pain and had alcohol in it and tasted bitter, it was called a "bitter." It don't take no rocket scientist to figure out how they got their name.

Bitters were much more popular in frontier times than many people realize. Names like Hostetter, Angostura, and Quaker were common household names to frontiersmen. Quakers the likes of Doctor Bill Crawford and Jim Ferdon sold their bitter tonics nationwide in traveling medicine shows during the waning days of the nineteenth century.

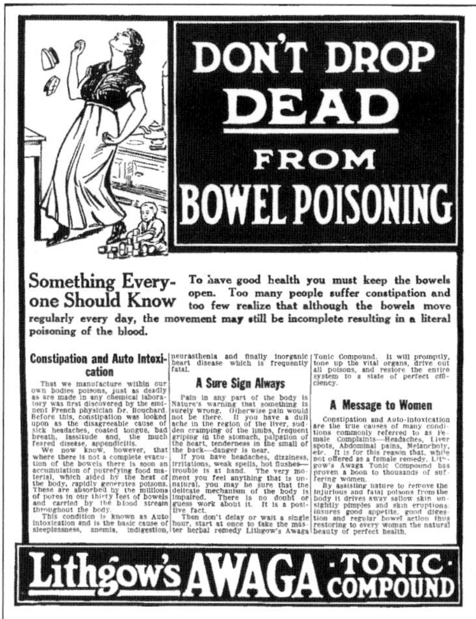


A tonic is an agent (as a drug) that increases body tone; one that invigorates restores, refreshes, or stimulates; as in a fluid-based preparation for the scalp or hair or a flavored beverage to be taken orally. Iron, quinine, and strychnine (IQS) in ethanol (drinking alcohol), were the base ingredients of many tonics and were used to treat practically everything that ailed the frontiersman. Save for the alcohol, tonics were not immediate acting; they worked by building the body up. The iron in them was ferrous sulfate, the good kind, and if taken long enough, it did help those who were anemic or had "low blood," as the old-timers used to say. Quinine was used to treat chills and fever and malaria, prevalent ailments back then. Strychnine (rat poison) was used in many old tonics as a stimulant. In large doses, it was indeed fatal, but in extremely small amounts, it rivaled caffeine as a mental booster. Unfortunately, the strychnine available in pioneer days was the unrefined, unstandardized kind, the best of all for rat poisons, but the worst of all for human consumption.

Compounded correctly, strychnine, iron, and quinine prepara-

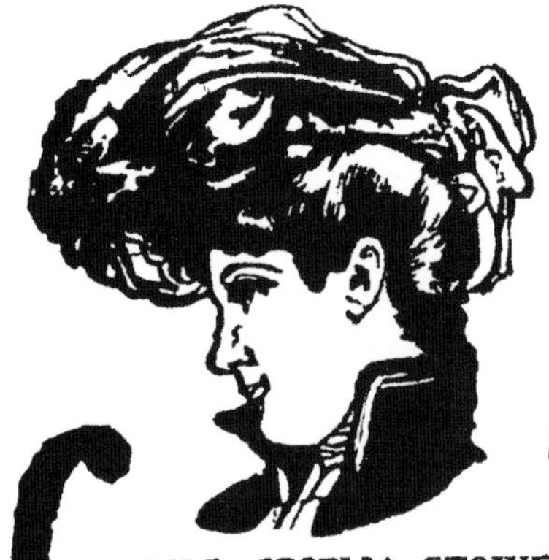

**MRS. CECELIA STOWE,**
Orator, Entre Nous Club.

176 Warren Avenue,
Chicago, Ill., Oct 22, 1902.

For nearly four years I suffered from ovarian troubles. The doctor inslated on an operation as the only way to get well. I, however, strongly objected to an operation. My husband felt disbeartened as well as I, for home with a sick woman is a disconsolate place at best. A friendly druggist advised him to get a bottle of Wine of Cardui for me to try, and he did so. I began to improve in a few days and my recovery was very rapid. Within eighteen weeks I was another being.

Cecelia Stowe

Mrs. Stowe's letter shows every woman how a home is suddened by female weaknes and how completely Wine of Cardui cures that sickness and brings health and happiness again. Do not go on suffering. Go to your druggist today and secure a $1.00 bottle of Wine of Cardui.

**WINE of CARDUI**

tions were quite effective. As often as not, though, they were altered with heavens knows what and sold in traveling sideshows as miracle cures. Adding 40 percent ethyl alcohol (ethanol or drinking alcohol) made the concoctions sell even better. The addition of alcohol fermented from grain made knowing who prepared it even more critical. An ill-prepared batch of tonic based on the old IQS formula could be a double-bladed sword not only because of the amount of strychnine in it but because as often as not the alcohol used was moonshine, and there is a thin line between good moonshine and bad. During the distilling process, the temperature at which wood alcohol (a deadly poison—the kind used to cook with in fondue pots) and ethyl alcohol (the drinking kind) came through the copper coils of crude stills was very close. What good did it do to cure chills and low blood if the patient went blind or died in the process?

## *Medicinal Waters and Wines*

Medicinal waters were used as early as the first century B.C. There are two types of medicinal waters: aromatic waters and mineral waters. *Aromatic waters* were solutions containing medicinal principles in the form of gasses or volatile oils (oils that evaporate on standing). They were distilled from either dry or fresh herbs. The principal portion of the oils was skimmed off, leaving a liquid that retained the taste and odor of the plant used. These steam-medicated waters, however, were unstable and spoiled rapidly. The process of triturating (rubbing into a powder) so as to divide the essential oils into minute particles and make them more soluble was accomplished by using pumice stone, magnesium carbonate, or silica (sand). This process produced more permanent solutions after being filtered. Previous to 1880, carbonate of magnesia was the medium used. Recovering the volatile oils from the solutions by adding them to olive oil, then adding potash, produced soap. Adding acid to the soap liberated the volatile oil.

The most popular medicinal aromatic waters were camphor water, menthol water, orange-flower water, rose water, fennel water, spearmint water, peppermint water, and lemon water. Camphor, peppermint, spearmint, and orange and lemon were used as carminatives (relieved intestinal gas and stomach pain) and as antiemetics. The others were mostly used as flavorings or vehicles for perfumed toilet waters or in other potions.

Mineral waters contained alkalis, metals, and gaseous or other substances (with or without salt) that had therapeutic value. The most popular contained salt, sodium carbonate, iron, sodium sulfate, magnesium, calcium, and sodium iodide. In combinations, the ingredient in excess determined its classification. Many were used as bases for tonics. There were several types: mineral acid waters, chalybeate waters, sulfur waters, saline waters, calcic waters, sea waters, alkaline waters, silicious waters, carbonated waters, and purgative waters, each varying in its effects on the body.

Acidic mineral waters were used for dyspepsia, dropsy, and gravel. Most *chalybeate waters* contained iron and were used to treat anemia, dyspepsia, gout, diabetes, and diarrhea. *Sulfur waters* were used as diuretics, for kidney stones, gout, rheumatism, and deranged conditions of the stomach and liver. *Saline waters* were used for chronic constipation, jaundice, gallstones, and renal irritability. *Calcic waters* were thought valuable in cystitis, diabetes, and dyspepsia.

*Sea water* was used as an emetic and purgative and as a bath to remove toxins from the body. *Alkaline waters* were antacid and diuretic. *Purgative waters*, in small doses, were laxatives; in large doses, they were cathartic in action. *Silicious mineral waters* were chiefly used in chronic affections of osseous and ligamentous structures. (Don't feel bad—I didn't know what *osseous* meant, either. The word just sounded good.)

*Carbonated mineral waters* were used in beverages and as antacids and for dyspepsia.

## *Lotions and Emulsions*

Lotions were watery solutions, suspensions or dispersions of medicaments intended for external application to the body. Early lotions were notorious for "falling out" or separating and had to be shaken before use. Boiled okra and aloe vera juices were used to make lotions smooth and help prevent settling. Emulsions were the internal lotions, soft liquid remedies usually the color of milk, prepared by mixing oily forms of oral medicines in water by means of tiny amounts of surfactant (soap), which stabilized the final product. They were harder to prepare but remained stable longer than lotions. An emulsion that settled out was said to "crack."

### *Pastes, Ointments, Poultices, Plasters, Oils, Liniments, Fats, Salves, and Rubs*

A medicinal paste is a standardized product of semisolid form that can be mucilaginous, or mixtures of starch, talc, or other dry products, which contains just enough water to soften without liquefying. Pastes are used as vehicles to carry drugs that are commonly applied topically. Though some may contain petroleum or fatty acids, most consist of a water base.

Balsams were oily, aromatic, resinous substances that flowed spontaneously from or by incision from certain trees and shrubs. They were considered to be any plant resin that healed, soothed, mitigated suffering, or ministered to the mind.

Ointments are mixtures of medicaments with fats, waxes, or hydrocarbons that are applied to the skin. Like pastes, they contain just enough emollients to remain solid without liquefying at room temperature. Unlike pastes, ointments commonly have melting points slightly above normal body temperature, and when applied, they liquefy to some extent to disburse the drug. Ointments usually leave a sticky, greasy look. Pastes tend more to coat and protect without liquefying.

Poultices are soft compositions of starch, bran, meal, flaxseed, or other suitable substances that are applied to the body to treat sores or inflamed areas. Poultices commonly contained rubefacients like capsicum, menthol, wintergreen, clove, iodine, or turpentine that, if left too long, reddened, blistered, or caused sloughing of skin.

Plasters, like poultices, contained medicating agents that were

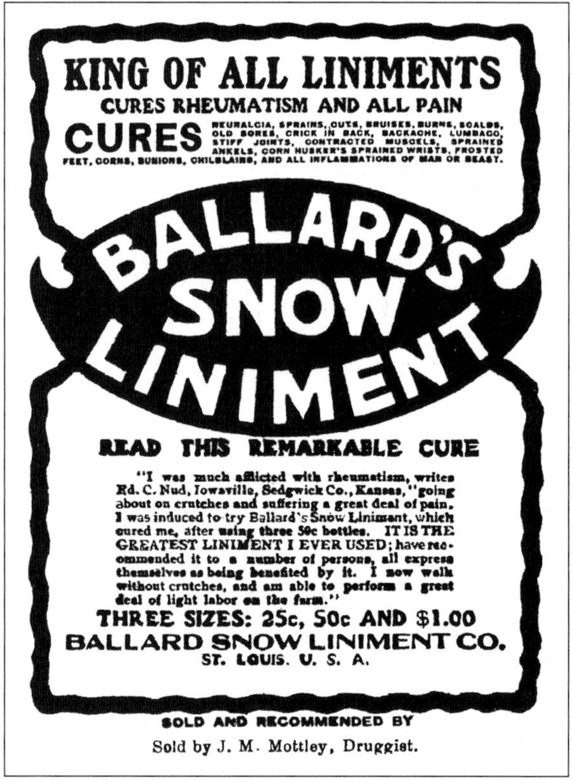


dispersed in pastelike vehicles. They were commonly covered with thin muslin, cloth, or other suitable wrap. The drugs they contained were not usually so strong as to be irritating if left on the skin for prolonged periods. Many plasters contained capsicum, urea, and camphor or other soothing agents. Back plasters are still commercially available in drug stores.

KING OF ALL LINIMENTS
CURES RHEUMATISM AND ALL PAIN
CURES NEURALGIA, SPRAINS, CUTS, BRUISES, BURNS, SCALDS, OLD SORES, CRICK IN BACK, BACKACHE, LUMBAGO, STIFF JOINTS, CONTRACTED MUSCELS, SPRAINED ANKELS, CORN HUSKER'S SPRAINED WRISTS, FROSTED FEET, CORNS, BUNIONS, CHILBLAINS, AND ALL INFLAMMATIONS OF MAN OR BEAST.
BALLARD'S SNOW LINIMENT
READ THIS REMARKABLE CURE
"I was much afflicted with rheumatism, writes Ed. C. Nud, Iowaville, Sedgwick Co., Kansas, "going about on crutches and suffering a great deal of pain. I was induced to try Ballard's Snow Liniment, which cured me, after using three 50c bottles. IT IS THE GREATEST LINIMENT I EVER USED; have recommended it to a number of persons, all express themselves as being benefited by it. I now walk without crutches, and am able to perform a great deal of light labor on the farm."
THREE SIZES: 25c, 50c AND $1.00
BALLARD SNOW LINIMENT CO.
ST. LOUIS. U. S. A.
SOLD AND RECOMMENDED BY
Sold by J. M. Mottley, Druggist.

Oils are divided into two classes, fatty oils and essential oils. *Fixed oils* are the same thing as *fatty oils* and differ from fats only as to their melting point—those that are liquid at room temperature are generally called fixed oils; those that are solid or semisolid at room temperature are generally called fatty oils. *Essential oils* differ from fatty oils in that they are volatile and are composed of naturally occurring biochemical products of plants. Examples of volatile oils are orange oil, peppermint oil, lemon oil, and rose oil.

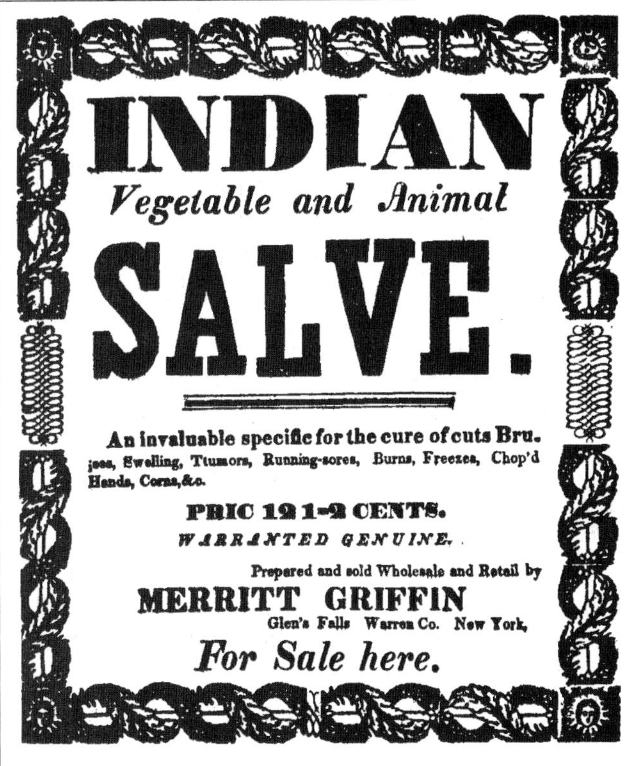


Cold-pressed essential oils are pressed hydraulically or squeezed from plants without the aid of heat.

Liniments are liquid preparations that are commonly activated by rubbing them on the skin. Most liniments used fixed aromatic oils, volatile oils, or alcohol and/or water combinations. Some liniments were prepared by mixing water into oil by adding water sudsed with lye soap or by adding limewater and shaking. Adding oils to ammonia water produced an oil-in-water emulsion. Liniments containing medicines and water alone were not as effective since they didn't seem to "penetrate" the body as well. Actually, many of the medicaments never penetrated at all; the alcohol or oils simply evaporated, leaving a cooling soothing effect. Water took too long to dry, and it just didn't smell "mediciney." Applying liniments with friction facilitated the action of a liniment simply because the physical movement itself released more of the drug at one time. If the liniment contained camphor or menthol or wintergreen, rubbing made it feel cooler, and therefore the liniment was much more effective as a cure-all.

A salve is any unctuous (smooth and greasy) substance that adheres to the skin and contains medications that soothe or heal. *Salve* is usually synonymous with *ointment*, except salves don't necessarily melt at body temperature; they retain their sticky, greasy integrity without dissolving or evaporating.

Salves contain medications dispersed primarily in waxy or petroleum bases, like the harder cerates and the thinner Vaseline-style products. Many salves contain aromatics that work by being inhaled, or they are applied to protect. The world's most famous rubbing salve is Vicks VapoRub, or Vicks salve, which originally was little more than camphor and menthol mixed in Vaseline. Salves make up many of the preparations used for chapped lips that protect as well as medicate and soothe.

## THE DRYS

### *Medicinal Folded "Powders"*

A powder is any dry substance composed of minute particles, either natural or artificial, that are comminuted or triturated into fine dustlike constituents. As many frontier drugs were available in powdered form, their dispensing and consumption by taking them directly were carried about more conveniently than by taking them in liquid forms.

Medicinal folded powders were individual doses carefully measured and dispensed in folded slick paper. These "powders" were easier to swallow than pills or tablets and were particularly suited for children and people who had difficulty swallowing. Being placed in liquids for long periods of time decomposed many drugs. For this reason, powders remained fresher for longer periods of time. Dumping them in juice or other palatable liquids immediately before taking made it easier for children and the elderly to take.

The major disadvantages of taking medicinal folded powders directly were that many vegetable- and mineral-based drugs were bitter and tasted bad. And since the medicines were usually opened and dumped directly onto the tongue to be taken, many people just didn't like taking them.

Some powdered drugs absorbed water from the air and if left exposed to heat, or allowed to get old, formed into hard or gooey masses.

Some drug combinations were even explosive. Oxidizing agents like potassium chlorate that were triturated (ground together) in a mortar with a reducing agent, like tannic acid, exploded, sometimes violently. Frontier druggists learned quickly that they had to pulverize these types of medicines separately; then gently mix them together without pressure—that or prepare the ingredients in separate folded papers with proper instructions, and let the patient mix them. The most common frontier drugs that exploded when put together were these:

- *Potassium chlorate and charcoal:* Potassium chlorate was used in frontier times as an antiseptic on skin and mucous membranes. Charcoal was used as an antacid and as an antidote for poisons.
- *Potassium nitrate and sulfur:* Potassium nitrate was used as a diuretic and as a topical antiseptic. Sulfur was used as a laxative, a diaphoretic, and a topical antiseptic.
- *Sodium peroxide and tannic acid:* Sodium peroxide liberated oxygen and was used for acne. Tannic acid was used as an astringent, as a treatment for burns, for sore throat, to harden the nipples of a nursing mother, for diarrhea, and to suppress mucosal weeping.
- *Silver nitrate and volatile oils:* Silver nitrate was used as a

caustic and as prophylactic treatment of babies' eyes for venereal disease. Volatile oils were oils like lemon, orange, peppermint, and lavender.

You didn't know that the old saying; "Boy, that was a blast!" came from taking and making frontier medicines, now, did you?

## *Pills*

Little round pills were perhaps the most popular form for taking dry medicinals in earlier times. Old prescription compounding books go into great length to describe pill-making processes and formulas, and considering the conditions and the times, the processes were quite technical. Elaborate mahogany and brass pill-making trays brought from abroad were used to make what were called "good" pills. The process became a true art form. Druggists were evaluated on their ability to produce consistent and standardized pills. This is where the nickname "pillroller" for a druggist comes from.

Medicaments were mixed into pasty masses, pressed, and rolled into little balls of all sizes, depending on the pill machine used. Some were simply rolled by hand, the amount of drug purely determined by trial and error. Many pills were coated with thin layers of sugar- or honey-based mixtures, some of which contained silver, mercury, and even gold. Little, round handheld canisters with removable tops called *pill treens* (precursors to the huge tumbling vats still employed today by drug companies) were used to coat pills. The process of coating a pill with metal was quite involved and required specialized equipment. Most people are familiar with the common mortar and pestle, the modern-day pharmacist's trademark.

Metals like silver and gold were melted and poured into iron mortars (specially designed bowls), which contained powdered chalk. The molten mass was then triturated (ground and reduced in size) with a metal pestle until it cooled. When the metal came in contact with the chalk, under continuous abrasion, as it cooled it so-

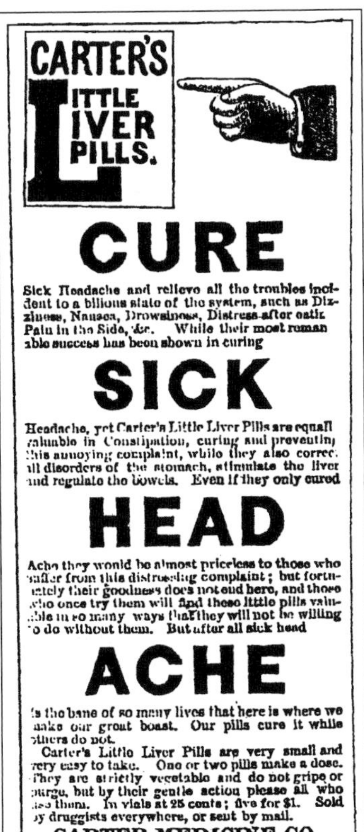


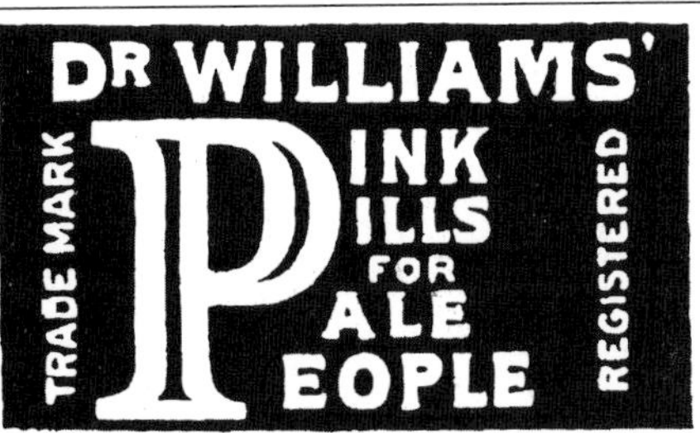


DR WILLIAMS' PINK PILLS FOR PALE PEOPLE ARE NEVER SOLD BY THE DOZEN OR HUNDRED, BUT ALWAYS IN PACKAGES. AVAILABLE AT ALL DRUGGISTS OR DIRECT FROM DR WILLIAMS MEDICINE CO. SCHENECTADY, N.Y., 50 CENTS PER BOX OR 6 BOXES FOR $2.50.

lidified into powderlike flakes. The chalk was removed, and the flaked metal was used to coat the pills. Flaking metal in powdered chalk required the used of heat-resistant mortars and pestles. Preheated porcelain mortars were later used with pestles that had wooden handles for easier mixing of the hot bowl's contents. Many of the older metal pestles had one rounded end and one flat and slightly concave end called a "clump buster," which was used to reduce lumps not only in molten metal preparations but in grinding clumpy herbals and lumpy powders. Pure glass and wooden mortars and pestles were used solely for mixing heat-sensitive preparations.

Some pills were coated with a silver and mercury combination.

This mixture became so hard that on occasion the pill passed completely through the body seemingly unaffected. Ironically, the coating released just enough mercury to have a laxative action. The pills were, on occasion, recovered, and reused. These silver mercury pills were called "booty balls."

Tablet triturates were small tablets made by molding soft sugar-based, alcohol-moistened masses. Very fine powders were required. These were the precursors to today's rapidly dissolving hypodermic tablets. Most tablet triturate machines were made of metal or hard rubber. The moist mass was spread into the mold's holes, a pressing cap was placed over it and pressure applied, and then the mass was ejected and allowed to dry. These hand molds were replaced later with elaborate, mechanized equipment that used dry powder, which was pressed out under extremely high pressure.

### *Cachets*

Cachets were crude precursors to capsules, the process of which came to us from Europe, particularly France. Flour was mixed into thick dough and rolled into thin sheets. Placed in molds, it was cut and fashioned into little concave circles that were dried. Powdered medications were placed in the hollows of one formed side. The edges were then moistened, and another side was placed over it. The cachets were then pressed together and allowed to dry to form an oyster-cracker-looking pill. The resulting wafer was dipped in water a moment to moisten it, placed on the tongue, and swallowed whole by chasing it with a glass of water. The commercially known Konseal machine was a modern kit used by doctors and druggists to make cachets from convenient premade components.

The primary advantage to taking cachets was the same as that of taking capsules today. The dose form floated and went down much easier; when swallowed, it didn't stick to the tongue or adhere to the back of the throat like a dry pill did.

THE

# "SIMPLE" PILL COATER,

SPECIALLY RECOMMENDED BY DR. SYMES,

*For Coating Small Quantities of Pills with Ease & Perfection.*

The almost universal demand for Coated Pills has brought prominently into use these Pill Coating Machines, which now find a place on most Dispensing Counters. The "Simple" Pill Coater will coat any quantity of Pills, from one dozen to a quarter-of-a-pound. For larger quantities we recommend the Rotary Machine which will coat any quantity, from a quarter to a pound.

## DIRECTIONS FOR USE—By DR. SYMES.

Dissolve ¼ oz. of Tolu (the resin left from preparing the Syrup answers well,) in 1 oz. Ether. Mark this Solution No. 1.

Mix equal parts of Syr. Mucilage and water, and mark Solution No. 2. Place the Pills to be coated in a pot and moisten the surface well with Solution No. 1, transfer quickly to a box containing a good supply of Levigated French Chalk, shake for half a minute, place the Pills in the Coater, and rotate rapidly, applying a gentle heat (the cover being off) for four or five minutes, remove from the source of heat, and continue the rotation a few minutes longer, set aside for an hour, and repeat the process, substituting Solution No. 2, and after the Pills have been set aside the second time, place the cover on the Coater and rotate rapidly for a few minutes, to give a final polish to the surface.

By this means a gross or two of Pills may be coated with the utmost facility.

N.B.—It is important that the Pills be hard and well-made.

The following unsolicited Testimonial is a sample of many others which we have received.

STOURBRIDGE,
Sept. 21st, 1881.

Gentlemen,

The Pill Coater answers admirably, my first attempt has produced a result quite equal to any of the Coated Pills I have ever bought, and the trouble is but slight.

Yours, &c.,
T. P. CLARK.

*A Complete Catalogue* OF *Druggists' Sundries* (*500 Illustrations*) *Sent Post Free to any part of the World on application.*

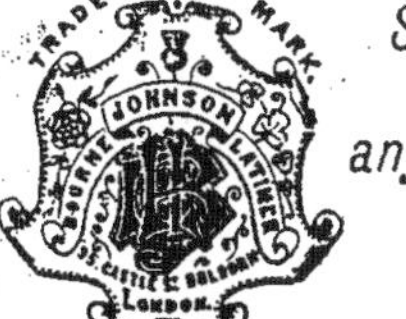


**35, CASTLE STREET, HOLBORN,**
**LONDON, E.C.**

### *Solid and Semisolid Extracts*

Often referred to as *draughts*, solid extracts were concentrated preparations obtained by evaporating solutions of vegetable and animal drugs with a suitable menstruum and adjusting the mass to equal five times stronger than fluid extracts. Often, the resultant mass exhibited a plastic consistency. Semisolid extracts were those more similar in consistency to thick molasses. Examples are black draught powder and extract of belladonna.

### *Effervescents*

Effervescents were granular dry preparations usually prepared with a bicarbonate powder base that fizzed when added to water. Many patent aperients (laxatives) were prepared in effervescent forms. A teaspoonful of the medicament was added to glass of water, allowed to bubble off, then taken. A still popular modern-day effervescent is Alka-Seltzer.

### *Sprinkle Powders, Sugartits, Talcs, and Insufflates*

Sprinkle powders, talcs, and insufflates were finely pulverized, dustlike medications that were prepared for both internal and external application. Medicinal topical dusting powders were applied as drying agents to treat ulcers and to prevent chafing, diaper rash, and saddle gauld. Insufflates were medicated dusting powders that were inhaled to treat asthma, catarrh, consumption, and emphysema.

Sugartits were prepared by cutting a soft piece of muslin or other clean cloth, pouring a small amount of granulated sugar or the dried and powdered granules from a molasses jar, forming a ball around the sugar with the cloth, and tying it tightly. Medications like laudanum, paregoric, or chloral in combination with a flavoring agent like lemon or the like were applied to the ball thus formed, and the baby was allowed to suck on it. As saliva dissolved the sugar, the medicine got swallowed and the baby got the medicine.

### *Lozenges, Troches, and Pastilles*

Lozenges and troches were convenient masses of therapeutic substances, which were designed to slowly dissolve in the mouth to give continuous application of a mild medicine to the mucous membranes of the mouth and throat. Potent, often disagreeable medicines could be masked in convenient, candylike dose forms and given to children.

The process involved making a hot mass, usually composed of a sugar base, rolling it into a sheet, cutting it with punches much like a cookie cutter, and allowing it to cool. The common cough drop (both troches and lozenges) were handmade this way.

Pastilles were soft varieties of troches and lozenges. They were usually transparent and were prepared in a base of acacia, sucrose, water, coloring, and flavoring.

### *Suppositories*

Frontier medical practice involved a lot of puking, bleeding, and crapping, but nothing was more disgusting, or humiliating, than the dreaded suppository. Enemas even had a slight edge over suppositories. The primary bases for suppositories in frontier times were cocoa butter and/or hard lard. The mass was gently heated, medication was added by stirring, and then the mass was cooled and rolled by hand into tubes, which were cut into convenient weighed doses or poured into molds and allowed to cool. Suppository molds came in all shapes and sizes. The trick to making good cocoa butter suppositories was not to heat the base too much. If it got too hot, it broke down the integrity of the solidifying texture and failed to solidify again. When gelatins came into use in the early twentieth century, suppositories were much more stable in warm climates and were particularly used to make "inserts," which are still popular today for vaginal and urethral medicine application.

I'll never forget the look on my old professor's face when he saw the first suppository I ever made. We were in dispensing lab on a

Friday afternoon, as I recall. He had given each student a different prescription for suppositories. On my order, he had mistakenly failed to put a quantity. I prepared my suppository mass as per instructions and went looking for him. He was nowhere to be found, so, I made one, humongous suppository by pouring the entire melted mass into a conical flask and letting it cool. When he returned, the whole class held their breaths and snickered in anticipation. Dr. Albers walked to the monstrosity sitting on the table, wiped his mouth with a leathered palm, looked at my prescription, at the suppository, up to me. A frown furrowed his brow before he said, "You did it right." He then smiled and gave me an A.

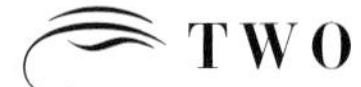 TWO

# *Treatments: The Good, the Sad, and the Ungodly*

MANY OLD MEDICINES and treatments were indeed pure bunk. However, out of some came the saving of a life. One cannot help but wonder how many really excellent remedies were buried with those who discovered and used them during America's earlier days. The following are stories and memorable encounters, some indeed good, some tragically sad, and some downright ungodly.

## FRONTIER VIAGRA

The inability to have sexual connections is as old as mankind. Many modern medications are notorious for exacerbating the problem. Old physician's manuals like doctor Frank Miller's book, *Domestic Medical Practice: A Household Adviser in the Treatment of Diseases for Family Use* (in its twenty-third edition in 1913), states that opium, tobacco, arsenic, nitrate of potassium, and bicarbonate of soda caused impotency. Dr. Miller had his own formula, which he touted in his book as being successful in treating it.

**Dr. Miller's Impotency Prescription**
Arsenious acid, one-fortieth grain
Sulfate of strychnine, one-thirtieth grain
Sulfate of quinine, one-half grain
Reduced iron, one-half grain
*Directions*: Make one hundred pills. Take one pill three times daily, after meals.

From a purely scientific standpoint, only two of the ingredients, iron and quinine, had any real medical significance. Two were potent poisons. The redundancy in his treatment is interesting when you consider that on the same page he boldly states that arsenic "causes" impotency and then puts it in his remedy. Maybe things haven't changed as much as we think. Today, women pick up and pay for as much Viagra for their husbands as their husbands do for themselves. Perhaps this formula served best those frontier women with ulterior motives.

Another outlandish cure in Miller's book relates to the good doctor's treatment of prostatitis. He expounds: "The prostate is a muscular body, normally about the size of a horse chestnut, surrounding the neck of the bladder and a part of the urethra. It is therefore a sexual organ. Inflammation may result from unnatural or prolonged sexual excitement, or from stricture."

My amusement, aside from his astounding declaration of what a male sexual "organ" happens to be, is what does "unnatural" sexual excitement mean? What, besides a woman, was a cowboy or a settler that close to back then? (Hey, they don't call 'em cowpokes for nothing . . . sorry!)

## MAMOIDES' APHORISMS

Don't get me wrong. I'm not an atheist. I unwind toilet paper off the roll like any other right-handed Christian. Spiritual healing has its place. Prayer does help. But some things spiritually professed healers and ancient physicians promoted, I must question. To me, foreplay has no business at a funeral.

In the sixteenth century, an alchemist/physician by the name of Paracelsus had the wonderful idea that a plant's structure was a clue to its medical use and helped determine its usefulness. Walnut meat resembled brain tissue and was thought to cure brain disease. Brightly colored flowers were good for the eyes; juicy plants aided nursing mothers. Figs were said to aid manhood. I love that image.

Old Paracelsus did take the right path when he introduced metals to his pharmacopoeia: iron, lead, copper, potassium, magnesium, and mercury, the building blocks of future medicines. But then along came Moses.

In his book, *The Medical Legacy of Moses Maimonides*, Fred Rosner relates, and I quote from page 66, "Mouse excrement, if pulverized in vinegar, is beneficial for alopecia (the loss of hair). The brain of a camel, if dried, prepared in vinegar and imbibed, is of value against epilepsy." And he goes on and on to relate the ridiculous benefits of lamb brains rubbed on the gums of teething children, the body cleansing benefits of pulverized earthworms, the eating of rabbit heads for treating tumors, and a lotion of sugar to strengthen vision. He expounds on the benefits of snakeroot, an aromatic, bitter stimulant, for use on hemorrhoids. How stimulating.

## MISS CLARE: LA YEGUA

Suicides were prevalent in early times, but frontier women didn't have ready access to sleeping pills as did Marilyn Monroe and some others. They did, however, have access to a clear, colorless, mobile liquid called chlorof (chloroform) that had a characteristic, ethereal odor and a burning sweet taste. Wood alcohol, the most poisonous of all alcohols, was also available.

His name was Frank Goodwyn. Nicknamed El Pinto Viejo by the Mexican element on the King Ranch, which meant "the Old

Paint," derived from the ancient paint horse he rode. The name was in no way complimentary, but he answered to it to get along.

The mighty King Ranch, one of America's earliest, had so many cowhands that it had its own schoolhouse and its own general store. At the Norias, the largest portion of the ranch, the ranch hands had built a schoolhouse, a small white box with a red roof, on a sandy hill. Teachers seldom remained at the ranch longer than a term or two. They either found another, better-paying job or married and moved on.

One spring day Frank, his mother, and a whole slew of students stood in anticipation, awaiting the arrival of the ranch's new schoolteacher, Miss Clare.

The rain had slowed to a soft pitter-patter on the day she arrived at the main house. Dressed in black, she hobbled briskly to the porch, stopped at the steps, flipped off her bonnet, and smiled upward toward the clouds. "My goodness, it feels so good. Lord knows we needed it." Head tilted, chin high, she stuck out her tongue lapping at the falling rain. "Isn't it wonderful?"

Frank's mother leaned to him and whispered, "My God. She's one-legged."

He looked up to his mother and then back to the teacher as all in attendance, straight-faced and solemn, removed their hats and tried to force a smile.

"Glad to have you in Norias," Mrs. Goodwyn said as she stepped forward and extended a hand.

Miss Clare bounced up the steps on two crutches, took Mrs. Goodwin's hand, and shook it. "Glad to be here," she replied and smiled.

Frank admired her from the start, her cordial demeanor and cheerful disposition and the way she moved about with such grace on that one high-heeled shoe and those crutches. When asked about how she'd lost her leg, Miss Clare paused a moment. The thought flickered a momentary frown across her eyes before she smiled and said, "I slipped on a rug and fell." And that was that. No one ever asked again. Norias was well known as a refuge for twisted and crippled spirits.

The Norias schoolhouse had a huge porch facing west and two windows on each side, no playground. Over the hill to the east stood the Mexican houses. The one-room house of learning was built between the Anglo and Mexican houses and connected the two cultures. The *vaquero* element on the ranch overwhelmed Miss Clare and the English she spoke. Ridiculed in Spanish but respected in her native tongue, she had her hands full from the beginning.

She tried to understand the crude Spanish the children spoke and listened intently trying to understand. The Mexican kids had no need to speak softly to ridicule without her knowing it. They named her *la yegua* (the mare). When a child got a paddling, they laughed and said the mare had up and thrown them. The whippings not only gave the vaquero children reason to dislike her; more important, when she paddled Frank, it gave him a sense of respect among his peers. But she never gave up trying to discipline and teach him or them.

A ranch hand once commented that the way Miss Clare hobbled made it hard to tell which leg was missing, a distinction that only became clear upon standing right before her. But even handicapped by her unduly twisted physique, she could do more on one leg than most could on one.

She was a magnificent storyteller. Late in the afternoons, she and Frank often sat on the horse fences beneath a wobbling windmill and made up stories about heroes and giants. Miss Clare would start a story and then let Frank continue it. They would laugh and enjoy each other's company for hours on end. She was the jolliest person Frank had ever known.

Miss Clare ran on those crutches and played tagball with him and the other students. She caught the ball as often as anyone and could catch even the swiftest of the other boys. She seemed to be trying extra hard to be happy. Yet, there were days when she got moody.

During the quiet times in class when everyone was reading or doing assignments, she'd take one of the many letters she carried from her purse and read. Frank sat quietly and watched as she blotted tears and sniffed. She'd look up and fight to compose herself and go on.

Everything went well until one day Miss Clare up and told Frank she was going away, never to come back. That night, after supper, she entered the kitchen, took a white bowl from the cabinet, and climbed the stairs to her room. Near midnight her crutches banged on the floor.

When she failed to come down the next morning, Frank followed his mother up the stairs and watched as she knocked on the door. To Frank's and Mrs. Goodwyn's surprise, Miss Clare had unlatched it sometime during the night and left it ajar. She always kept it closed and locked.

The small-framed schoolteacher lay on her bed with a beautiful quilt pulled over her head. A note on the table beside her read, "Mrs. Goodwyn: Please don't let them take my body home. I want to be buried here near Norias."

Miss Clare planned her suicide well: filled the bowl with cotton, poured chloroform over that, drank a full bottle of wood alcohol, and then rammed her face into the damp cotton mess. She used a cardboard box carefully fashioned and prepared earlier to hold the bowl on her face after she passed out.

She related to Frank once that her favorite song was "Climbing Up the Stairs." She never really made it up the stairs to her true heaven. Her father refused to let her be buried at Norias. He insisted that the ranch hands ship her body back to San Antonio, where she was buried. (21–p. 86)

## SOFIE HERZOG: THE "BULLET SURGEON"

The first surgeons in pioneer days were barbers, and the first doctors and nurses were mothers. From aunts to grandmothers,

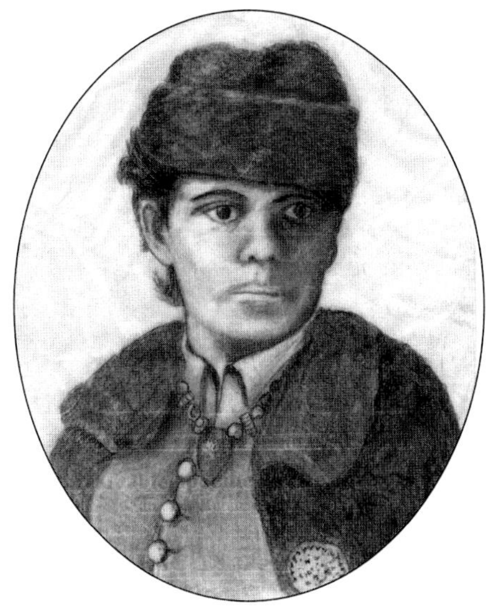

*Sofie Herzog, M.D. (1848–1925), the "Texas Bullet Surgeon," first lady physician in Texas*

midwives to wet nurses, women carried the burden on their slender shoulders of healing others. Many women who came west to the desolate prairies gave birth in covered wagons or in sod houses or under no roof at all. Young mothers, most no more than babies themselves, died during delivery or of loneliness; all who came west suffered. Frontier women, like our own mothers, worked hard raising their families, many doing so while their husbands plowed fields or rode horseback all day to eke out a living from the harsh lands of hope. Single-handedly mothers fought scurvy, malnutrition, whooping cough, croup, infection, colic, and high fever. Those stoic enough to come west carried the hopes of future generations in their wombs. Tragically, they left their own trails of tears. Tiny headstones dot pioneer cemeteries. Heaven only knows how many infants were buried with no markers. What frontier mother wouldn't have given a significant body part for a bottle of today's premixed penicillin or a plain old bottle of liquid Tylenol?

The town of Brazoria, Texas, like many frontier towns, was in dire need of someone to treat their ill and ailing. Brazoria's 1893 inhabitants were in a beehive of activity awaiting the arrival of their new physician, the first for Brazoria. Thick woods, marshes, and bottomlands nearby offered cover to many a cowboy of ill repute. The dreadful Texas heat, poor economic conditions, and short tempers made for regular gunfights. Malaria, yellow fever, snakebites, alligators, and other rough-country varmints plagued the brave people who lived there. They needed someone to treat their bullet wounds and heal them. Having its own doctor spoke highly of any town back then. And this was a "real" one, a certified and registered physician with papers to prove it, and he was coming here all the way from New York City.

What the good citizens of Brazoria got, much to their surprise, was a frontier version of Dr. Quinn, Medicine Woman—yes, a woman, if that don't beat all.

At a time when respectable womenfolk wore their hair long and in a bun, Dr. Sofie, as she came to be known, cut her hair short. This in no way inferred a gender preference, as it might be taken today. During her stay in Brazoria, Sofie gave birth to fifteen babies, including three sets of twins.

The "Medicine Woman" of Brazoria was as tough as they come—had to be. Even with her medical expertise, eight of her own died in infancy. In the 1880s, the life expectancy of a female was forty-four years. Sofie Herzog lived to be seventy-nine. She had a strong will and was a woman perfectly comfortable with horsehair in her belly button lint. She was well known, too, for her forceful personality.

Her practice depended on skillful surgical procedure and medicines of the day: castor oil, quinine, calomel, mustard plasters, and morphine. Bloodletting was a common treatment in her practice. She not only used whiskey and opium but heated that poker of hers and used it to cauterize bullet holes; that or dabbed pine tar or petroleum jelly mixed with gunpowder into the bullet hole, which was then ignited—a common practice in those days. Dr. Sofie wasn't at all adverse to taking that poker and properly attending to those who disagreed with her, either. She used leeches in her practice, too, leeches she gathered herself from local streams.

Medical practice in the late nineteenth century wasn't for the faint at heart. Her instruments included not only that poker but also saws for amputations, pliers for extracting teeth, and many other ghastly tools invented by the devil. She no doubt made use of a clyster syringe to give enemas with, the wash of which contained various herbal concoctions.

She became most famous for her expertise in removing slugs from slower cowboys. The bullets she removed she had made into a necklace, which she wore around her neck for good luck. Sofie was an avid outdoorsman, hunter, and a collector. Specimens of all kinds decorated her home: alligators, two-headed snakes in jars, a two-headed baby.

One of her last requests was to be buried in her "good luck" bullet necklace. Her children saw to her wishes with the morbid piece of jewelry, but they donated many of her human specimens and body parts to a state medical school. Her hides and other trophies were buried elsewhere.

Gunpowder was tried as an oral medicine during the nineteenth century, mixed with castor oil it was used as an emetic/cathartic, but the therapeutic threshold was too close to the toxic level. For several days after taking it, you had to be very careful which way you pointed either end. (14–p. 165; 17–accessed July 25, 2002; 19–p. 9)

## BAD MEDICINE

Aside from removing bullets and treating bullet holes, another gruesome problem many frontiersmen faced was treating puncture wounds from arrows. Compared to modern-day bows with their eccentric wheels, laminated graphite, fiberglass limbs, and Kevlar bowstrings, the dynamics of the bows the Indians used were puny by comparison. A standard compound bow used in hunting today can fling a 450-grain, razor-tipped, graphite composite arrow upward of 350 feet per second. That much weight, even traveling at such a seemingly slow speed when compared to a bullet, has enough energy to pass completely through, rib bones and all, a standard whitetail deer, elk, or man. The straight-limbed bows and crude arrows used by American Indians, though powerful enough to bring down a buffalo, didn't do it easily. Unless the projectile was driven straight into the heart (which seldom occurred), it took many more arrows to kill than one might suspect; and even then, the victim's demise was agonizingly slow.

A letter written by a soldier in the U.S. Calvary in 1867 illustrates. In the P.S. section of his correspondence, John L. McElhaney, Second U.S. Calvary, Fort McPherson, Nebraska Territory, writes to his brother:

> Since finishing the above [letter], I have secured another arrow which I enclose. The cuts are marked that you may place the pieces together again as they were originally. It is one of the one hundred and twenty five taken from the body of one man. It is the arrow of the Cheyenne's. The color of the paint about the feathers determines the tribe to which the arrow belongs. The red stains are human blood; the catch on the bowstring is broken. It, however, imperfect, as it is, will be a curiosity to you and many of the frequenters of the Shades.

Good straight arrows were an extremely valuable commodity to the American Indian. Indians used the bow and arrow to provide food. A good provider was well respected among his peers. The pride of losing an arrow into an enemy was counted as a coup and brought even more respect. In Indian society, an arrow could be used for no greater purpose.

As McElhaney mentioned, the color and markings on an arrow determined the tribe. He reports that the arrow had red on it that was probably blood. A Texas Comanche Indian has convinced me that the red most likely wasn't blood at all and that a common coloring for Plains Indians, particularly on the shaft and near the feathers (a primitive form of cresting), came from an insect known as the cochineal bug that lives to this day on the prickly pear cactus that festers southern landscapes. This little beetle harbors a brilliant red residue, which was used on arrows and in decorative Indian art. The bug spins a fuzzy web resembling a puff of cotton stuck to the face of cactus lobes. The beetles were carefully scraped off. When mashed, a brilliant red liquid exudes. Since old blood oxidizes and turns black within hours, I'm convinced that that the red McElhaney mentions wasn't blood but instead was cochineal remains.

Other colorings used by American natives were yellow sulfuric residues found naturally in dirt and sand and any other brilliant substance readily available. These colorings, along with the sinew from dead deer and buffalo used to attach arrowheads to arrows, as well as aconite, a poison derived from a plant, were occasionally applied to the tips. Indians were known on occasion to dip their arrow tips in the putrid juices of a decaying animal so as to pass the "death spirit" onto their enemy. The old, "push it through and break off the tip" method of removing an arrow exposed the victim to even more bad medicine and meant certain death and prolonged agony.

Contagion from the ground-up bugs and the bad medicine of death made these unclean arrows as deadly as bullets. Forcing a red-hot poker along the path of a bullet or arrow hole was a gruesome means of cauterizing and sterilizing the wound, but in many cases it did the job. (44–accessed April 3, 2001)

## AN UNEASY DOSE TO SWALLOW: THE STORY OF SERGEANT CHARLES FLOYD

Meriwether Lewis paused on his way to check on a sick soldier when he saw his partner, William Clark, sitting on a log beside the creek. William had his head down and his hands deep inside his pants in front.

"I'm afraid to ask what you're doing," Meriwether said, laughing.

William didn't look up or smile; his attentions were focused on his crotch, his fingers working daintily to pinch something from a tender, major body part. "Darned queer tick," he said. "He got me in the worst possible place, the very tip. I gotta get the head out, or it might fester like the one on my leg did."

Meriwether leaned to see better and snickered. "How do you know it's not a she tick?"

William looked up at Meriwether, down, up again, and grinned. Meriwether chuckled then added, "If this one swells like the tick bite on your leg did, you'll have every native woman around here chasing you."

They laughed in unison as William scratched, adjusted himself, and stood. It was then that Sergeant Patrick Gass came running to Meriwether's side. Gass's eyes went to William Clark's opened pants, and he stared a moment as if he'd forgotten what he came to say. William promptly tucked and buttoned.

"What is it, sergeant?" Meriwether asked.

"It's Floyd, sir; he's taken a turn for the worse."

Meriwether hurried along behind Clark to the ailing man's side and stared as his partner knelt to check the ashen-faced soldier's pulse. William looked up from a squawlike squat and said, "Mr. Cass, bring me my bag."

"Yes, sir."

"What are you going to do?" Meriwether asked.

"Nothing to do but give him some of Dr. Rush's pills."

"He's so loose now he's passing clear water."

"Yeah, I know, but whatever is causing his pain has got to be pushed on out of his body."

"Here, sir," Gass said, holding up a leather bag.

Meriwether took it from Gass's hand and began fumbling inside. He removed a small bottle and looked down at William. "How many?"

"Two." William had no sooner said that than the ailing man cried out in agonizing pain. "Better make it five," he said.

Meriwether watched then as William coaxed Floyd into swallowing the pills and chasing them with a small sip of water. Twice more the sergeant cried out before he finally relaxed. William Clark wiped Floyd's face with a damp cloth. Every time the poor man moaned Meriwether sensed a bit of pain in William's eyes.

Less than an hour passed before, of a sudden, young Sergeant Charles Floyd curled up into a ball, screamed loud enough to be heard back in Washington, and went limp all over.

By now, the men had gathered all around. William examined Floyd, checked his pulse at the wrist and neck, and raised a limp eyelid. With sad eyes, he looked up to Meriwether and said softly, "I'm afraid he' s gone."

Sergeant Charles Floyd was the only man to die on the Lewis and Clark expedition, a rather phenomenal occurrence considering the time and conditions under which the expedition took place. Only one death becomes even more astounding when you realize that there were no trained physicians on the trip. Floyd being diagnosed with a ruptured appendix is pure conjecture, too. His death having been hastened by a megadose of purgatives is also based on speculation. However, even though none of Floyd's drug treatments were documented in the Lewis and Clark journals, given the customary use of purgatives and bleeding, the chances are that such treatments were administered. If Floyd did have appendicitis, he would likely have died anyway. A purgative dose of Dr. Rush's pills would have surely and painfully hastened his demise.

There is also a consensus of interpretation as to the cause of Captain William Clark's illness at Three Forks for which he himself took five of Dr. Rush's pills. His having contracted a debilitating case of tick fever seems to be the most likely scenario. Clark's having himself taken such a large dose of purgatives strengthens the theory of the gruesome death of Sergeant Charles Floyd. When we study the fossil remains of history by reviewing old diaries and accounts, we find ourselves assuming a lot. As to whether William Clark got a tick on the tip of his . . . personality, well, I can't prove he actually did, but can anyone prove he didn't?

As per a list purchased for the trip that lasted from 1803 to 1806, the following is:

**The Contents of Meriwether Lewis and William Clark's Medicine Chest**

*15 pounds of powdered Peruvian bark (1753–1955).* Also known as cinchona. Used to treat auge (malaria) and to make bitters and tonics to treat fever and pain. Often mixed with gunpowder into poultices for snakebites and gunshot wounds.

*0.5 pounds of powdered Jalap (1753 to date).* Used as a cathartic and diuretic. Aided digestion by stimulating bile flow.

*0.5 pounds of powdered rhubarb (1753 to date).* Used as a laxative, as a stomachic for distension, and in ointments as an astringent for irritations and swelling tissue.

*4 ounces of powdered Brazilian ipecac (1753 to date).* Used as an emetic and expectorant. Mixed with opium powder (to make Dover's powder), it acted as a diaphoretic. Often used in tonics with iron.

*2 pounds of cream of tartar (1753 to date).* Potassium bitartrate. Used as a diuretic and laxative and in baking.

*2 ounces of camphor gum (1753 to date).* A soothing irritant for ointments—chapped lips, colds—and used in salves for respiratory distress. Applied topically for inflamed joints, rheumatism, and sprains. Taken internally in very small amounts (less than a pinch), it provided warmth and comfort to the gut, and its expectorant action stimulated the respiratory system and improved circulation. It was a stomachic and carminative.

*1 pound of asafoetida (1753–1960).* Taken orally, it was used as a stomachic, carminative, and flavoring. Externally it was used in enemas and poultices.

*0.5 pounds of gum of raw opium (700 A.D. to date).* The dried milk from poppies. Use for pain and rest, as an antispasmodic for urinary tract ailments, and for diarrhea.

*0.25 pounds of tragacanth (1753 to date).* Thickening agent used as an excipient for pill making and as a thickening agent for pastes, poultices, and plasters.

*6 pounds of sal glauber–sodium sulfate (1753 to date).* Glauber's salt was frontier Epsom salt. Taken orally as a saline laxative. Applied topically as an astringent soak for infection, aches, bruises, and sprains.

*2 pounds of saltpeter (1753 to date).* Potassium nitrate. A diuretic/diaporetic used for sunstroke and to dampen the craving for sex. Mixed into a paste, it was applied to the hollows of cavities in teeth to relieve pain.

*2 pounds copperas-ferrous sulfate (1753 to date).* Also known as green vitriol, ferrous sulfate was used as a tonic and an astringent in liniments.

*4 ounces laudanum (700 A.D. to date).* Used for pain and restlessness and diarrhea.

*6 ounces of sacchar, saturn (sugar of lead or acetite of lead) (1753 to date).* Used to make eyewashes, in penis flushes for gonorrhea, on bruises, and for diseases of the skin like eczema and psoriasis—any and all skin irritations. Acetite of lead decomposed readily in water and had to be made fresh. It was often saturated on a cloth or mixed with bread and applied as a compress.

*4 ounces of calomel, mercurous chloride (1753 to date).* Used as a purgative and for syphilis treatment.

*1 ounce of tartar emetic (1753 to date).* Potassium tartrate, emetic, expectorant in smaller doses. Laxative, diuretic. Applied to boils and infected skin abrasions.

*4 ounces of white vitriol (zinc sulfate) (1753 to date).* Used in eyewashes and in tonics and as an astringent.

*½ pound of columba rad (1753 to date).* Dried root of columba. Use as tonic. For diarrhea and as a bitter for dyspepsia and indigestion.

*¼ pound of elixir vitriol (1753 to date).* Ethylsulfuric acid. Astringent, stomach problems.

*2 pounds unquentum basilic flavoring compound of pine resin.* A combination of yellow beeswax and lard, for use as ointment base and for making salves. Probably hog lard, beeswax, and pine resin used for eczema, ringworm, jock itch, "gauld," and skin irritations.

*1 pound unquentum calimin.* A combination of ferric oxide and calamine ore, which contained zinc silicate and iron carbonate. Mixed into a paste, it was a good drying agent used for oozing sores caused by excoriations from poison ivy, the bites of mosquitoes, chiggers and other insects, and sun- or windburn.

*1 pound unquentum epispastric (also spelled* epispastic*).* A pyrotic blistering agent. Probably a mercurial like *Mercurius sublimatus corrosivis*, a sublimative corrosive that was used during the period.

*1 emplastic diachylon.* A plaster made from diachylon simple-lead oxide, in oil or glycerin for burns, wounds, and abrasions. Might possibly have been used as stomach plaster for liver ailments or maybe even as a styptic.

*¼ pound essence of menthol.* Used as a carminative, flavoring agent, expectorant, and decongestant for colds and as a cooling additive to plasters and pastes.

*¼ pound balsam of copaiboe.* Used for genital-urinary disinfectant, as a diuretic, stimulant, expectorant, and laxative. Aromatic, diaphoretic.

*¼ pound balsam of traumatopyra compound tincture of benzoin.* For abrasions, as an inhalant for bronchial irritations and asthma, and to toughen blisters.

*2 ounces magnesia.* Laxative, antacid to make milk of magnesia.

*1 pound of mercuriale.* For use in ointments for syphilitic lesions and for parasites and as a germicide.

*Borax (10 A.D. to date).* Used for catarrh (inflammation of the nasal and mucous membranes). Combined with glycerin it was applied as an anti-inflammatory for skin irritations and in shampoos. In a saturated solution, it was used as eyewash and as a mouth rinse for inflamed gums. Though poison, borax, in small doses, was taken for headaches.

*Flowers of sulfur (1753 to date).* Mixed with oils and ointments, it was used as an antifungal. Mixed with mercuriale ointment, it was used as a germicide and as treatment for mite infestations (parasites), such as scabies and cooties. Dusted on legs and boots, it repelled chiggers and ticks.

*Symple diachylon (two sticks).* Since a simple diachylon was made up of various plant juices and hardened exudates mixed in oil, this was probably a form of lip balm.

*600 pills Dr. Rush's prescription* of jalap and calomel purgative pills. Rush's pills, called "thunder bolts," contained fifteen grams of calomel and fifteen grams of jalap.

*2 ounces cloves (1753 to date).* For toothache, as flavoring, and as a carminative and stomachic.

*4 ounces cinnamon (1753 to date).* Used to make cinnamon water, which was used as a vehicle for Peruvian bark. Also used as a carminative, for dyspepsia, and as a tonic.

*Blistering ointment (1 pound).* Used as a pyrotic and rubefacient.

Lewis and Clark also carried assorted other medicinal equipment—a clyster enema syringe, several penis syringes, and bloodletting instruments. (7–p. 170; 13; 15; 27–p. 13)

## DIATHERMY: THE STORY OF HARRY EATON STEWART, M.D.

Dr. Harry Eaton Stewart didn't invent this darned contraption that sent high-frequency electricity through the human body; a man named Nikola Tesla did. Tesla studied the theory that heat could be induced in the body by bombarding it with high-frequency (low-amperage) electric current. A Frenchman named Jacques Arsene d'Arsonval experimented with Tesla's theory by sticking electrodes from a crude generator to the opposite the sides of a rabbit's leg. He proved that even though the skin outside wasn't hot, the meat was cooked inside, and hence heat was produced, and heat was well known to belay infection. The body's first defense against infection is to elevate its own temperature. This heating through with electricity became called *diathermy*.

Dr. Stewart let that "heat inside" theory mull around in his mind for a long time, and finally he mused that a controllable current might be practical. Was this quackery, or was it practical medicine?

Colonel George B. Young, of the United States Marine Hospital on Staten Island, New York, had previously asked Stewart to do something about the alarming rate of deaths caused by an epidemic of pneumonia spreading among his men. Together, Stewart and Young decided to give diathermy treatment a go.

Stewart remained skeptical, but he kept thinking about the mustard plasters and onion poultices commonly used to contain the fever that developed inside these sick people's lungs. It took him a while to convince himself to try it. Heck, it couldn't be any worse than onions. Was not this electricity a mere heat-producing poultice in itself?

He chose a man diagnosed with pneumonia who had no hope of survival. The soldier's relatives had already been notified, and his coffin ordered. Stewart placed the electrodes to the front and back of the sailor's chest and threw the switch. The machine hummed

# The Morse High Grade Office Electric Belts

Trade Mark Patented and Registered "MIOxRISE" Win Golden Opinions.

## STYLES.

No. 1 Belt—Full power, 24-cell double circuit belt, 2 batteries of 12 cells each. Standard belt for general use. Polished copper batteries and scarlet all wool ladies' cloth pockets. Made for ladies or gents.......... Per dozen.... $12 00

No. 2 Belt—Same as No. 1, cut with 4 anodes.......... Per dozen.... 12 00

No. 3 Belt—Single circuit, extra power, one continuous battery of 21 cells, long conducting cord for extremities. This belt is for severe cases of rheumatism or paralysis. Polished copper batteries and wool pockets...... Per dozen.... 12 00

No. 4 Belt—Same as No. 2, but finer extra silk, satin pockets, nickel plated batteries and all wire connections are heavily silver plated. Ladies or gents.......... Per dozen.... 15 00

No. 5 Belt—Same as No. 2 Belt, except the batteries are made of metal resembling aluminum. It generates as strong a current as the No. 2 Belt. Silk pockets; ladies or gents.......... Per dozen.... 9 60

No. 6 Belt—Single Circuit, 19 cells, in assorted colors plush pocket, with 3 anodes on belt and 2 on the elastic strap; gents. This is one of the showiest belts we make.......... Per dozen.... 12 00

No. 6 Belt—Single circuit, 14 cells, in fancy satin pocket, with 2 anodes on belt and 2 on the elastic strap. For ladies... Per dozen.... 12 00

No. 7 Belt—which is the No. 6 Belt complete, with lung and chest appliance which carries the current to 2 anodes on the chest and two on the back.......... Per dozen.... 24 00

Nos. 1, 2, 4, 5, 6 and 7 Belts have either the suspensory attachment or ladies' attachment as ordered.

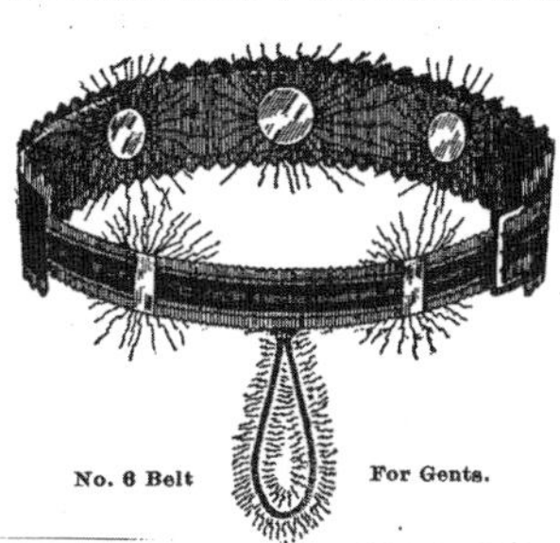

No. 6 Belt For Gents.

Long Conducting Cords can be used on any of the Morse High Grade Electric Belts in ordinary cases of Rheumatism, Paralysis and Neuralgia. Price 25c each. Cathode on the end of the cord is 1½ inches in diameter, solid nickel, highly polished; will reach from belt to top of head or sole of the foot. Extra attachment for leg or arm, with long conducting cord to be attached to any of the Morse High Grade Electric Belts. Price, 35c each. Ditto Head Bands, 35c each.

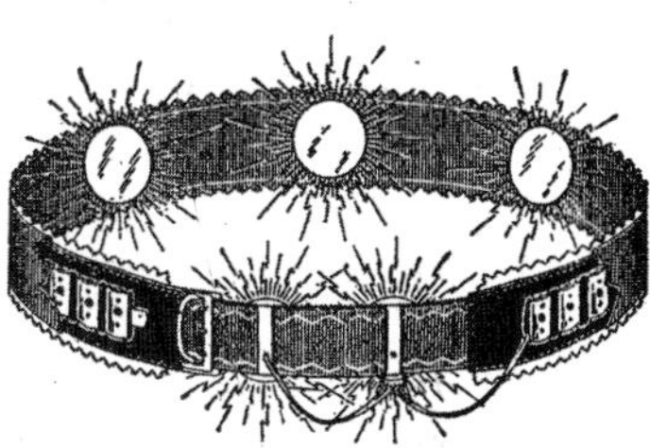

Cut of No. 6 Belt, Showing Battery.

No. 8 Belt—Single circuit, one continuous battery of 19 cells, extra strong 1¾ inch wide polished, nickel plated cells; 3 anodes on belt and 1 on the strap with suspensory attachment.......... Per dozen.... 18 00

No. 9 Belt—For Gents, single circuit, one continuous battery of 22 cells, 1½ inches wide, polished, nickel plated; 4 anodes on belt, 1 on strap and suspensory attachment. Pockets made of fine Scotch plaid silk or satin, specially made for us. Battery can be made with alternate nickel and copper cells if preferred.......... Per dozen.... 18 00

No. 10 Belt—For Ladies, similar to Gents' No. 9 Belt, but has ladies' attachment of 2 anodes on strap and 4 anodes on the pocket. This battery can be made with alternate nickel and copper cells if preferred.......... Per dozen.... 18 00

No. 11 Belt—Double pocket and battery quadruple strength, battery 2 inches wide and has 27 cells, 2 of such batteries to a belt. Pocket has 6 anodes on back and 2 on the strap. Most powerful Electric Belt made. Can be had for either lady or gent. With lung and chest attachment.......... Per dozen.... 48 00
Without lung and chest attachment.......... Per dozen.... 36 00

thirty thousand volts through the poor man's lungs. After the treatment, Stewart wasn't very hopeful and went home.

The next morning, on entering the ward, he was amazed to find the sailor sitting up in bed, reading. The pain behind the poor man's eyes was gone, and he was breathing much easier. Nine more soldiers were brought in for diathermy treatment. Only one died during the experiment; the norm was 50 percent. Many more times Stewart saw the "blue lips of death" turn pink after diathermy. Yet, he remained cautiously skeptical. Would these patients have recovered anyway? Still, his success with the new treatment continued, and so did his caution. It seemed that every case spoke better of it. One patient response impressed him more so than the others, a case of a comatose little boy who totally recovered after diathermy. Then there was a rich banker with diabetes and several other ailments that shouldn't have recovered but did. Was this really a blessing or a creeping joke in disguise? More and more patients responded, and soon, Dr. Harry Eaton Stewart became famous among his peers.

Paul De Kruif, who originally told this story in the *Ladies Home Journal* (1935: 27), closed the article by saying, "Then it's exactly as if we, as citizens, on account of the expense of it, would allow our fire departments to respond to alarms for the more severe kinds of fire. Expecting that then it would be unusually only property endangered, while in pneumonia it's human life."

History is packed with wonderful old success stories like this, with people like Dr. Henry Stewart who discovered a new treatment but was never able to convince the world of its usefulness. Had he had Oprah Winfrey or Larry King to extol his success, his name might to this day be deposited in our memories right up there beside Louis Pasteur, Thomas Edison, and the Wright brothers.

Electricity is used today to treat various forms of pain. A transcutaneous electrical nerve stimulation (TENS) unit, which requires a prescription, finds use to treat not only pain but also snake and insect bites, especially brown wood spider bites. It is thought that the current breaks down venom. (7–p. 373; 28–p. 18)

## HAVE A SEAT: BEN FRANKLIN'S "ELECTRISED" EXPERIMENT

We've all heard the story about the kite and lightening striking the key in Benjamin Franklin's hand back in 1752. Aside from that stupid trick, and the first parting of one's hair, Franklin's lesser heard of "scientific" contribution to society was another experiment with electricity—as a medicine.

In a letter to Sir John Pringle, a British physician (1707–1782), Ben Franklin relates that after hearing about the successful use of electricity as a medicine in Europe, several patients were brought to him from the Pennsylvania countryside to be "electrised," as he called it. Reportedly, he placed his patients on a stool wired to electric current and pulled the lever. He observed that the sparks generated an instantaneous sense of warmth and a definite increase in strength. Amazing. He also states that his patients gained immediate voluntary control of previously paralyzed extremities and had tingling sensations afterward. He boldly goes on to inform the good Dr. Pringle that his experiments with electricity were a failure. He writes in his letter to the doctor:

> Perhaps some permanent advantage might have been obtained if the electric shocks had been accompanied with proper medicine and regimen, under the direct supervision of a skillful physician. It may be, too, that a few great strokes [shocks], as given in my method, may not be so proper as many small ones; since, by the account from Scotland of a case, in which two hundred shocks from a phail were given daily, it seems a permanent cure has been made.

(A *phail* was a much weaker, handheld unit used by physicians in Europe, which wasn't too dissimilar from the one used by Dr. Stewart in his diathermy treatments.)

Ben Franklin not only discovered the Einstein hairdo but, apparently, a new means of dealing with criminals. No records were available as to what became of his "electrised" patients.

As early as 1800, records show that a Dr. Archibald Currie of Richmond offered an electric machine for use for medical purposes, which was designed to treat, successfully, hitherto incurable cases of paralysis, deafness, and even blindness. (7–p. 373)

## BEN FRANKLIN'S FAMOUS "TURPENTINE PILL"

Foolishness is always more fun when contrasted. The old "light against dark" has always been an artistic ploy to help make something, or someone, stand out. Forrest Gump was right; you never know what you're gonna get till you get into it. The original purpose of this story was to explore the foolishness of a famous founding father, Ben Franklin. Rumor had it he promoted the use of turpentine, in pill form, to make bowel gas smell better. Old Ben did indeed recommend the use of a turpentine pill to make farts not only smell better but to smell like violets, no less.

Here are some excerpts from Ben's response to the Royal Academy of Brussels, a body of Englishmen who had made some suggestions as to America's stance on freedom:

> It is universally well known, that in digesting our common food, there is created or produced in the bowels of human creatures, a great quantity of wind. That the permitting this air to escape and mix with the atmosphere, is usually offensive to the company, from the fetid smell that accompanyes it. . . . He that dines on stale flesh, especially with much addition of onions, shall be able to afford a stink that no company can tolerate; while he that has liv'd for some time on vegetables only, shall have the breath so pure as to be insensible to most delicate noses; and if he manage so as to avoid the report, he may anywhere give vent to his griefs, unnoticed. But there are many to whom an entire vegetable diet would be inconvenient, and a little Lime thrown into a Jakes will correct the amazing quantity of fetid air arising from the vast mass of putrid matter contain'd in such places, and render it rather

pleasing to the smell, who knows but what a little powder of Lime (or some other thing equivalent) taken in our food, or perhaps a glass of lime water drank at dinner, may have the same effect on the air produced in and issuing from the bowels? Certain it is also that we have the power of changing by slight means the smell of another discharge, that of our water. A few stems of asparagus eaten, shall give our urine a disagreeable odour; and a pill of Turpentine no bigger than a pea, shall bestow on it the pleasing smell of violets. And why should it be thought more impossible in nature, to find means of making perfume out of our wind than our water?

. . . The knowledge of Newtons Mutual Attraction of the particles of matter, can it afford ease to him who is rack'd by their mutual repulsion, and the cruel distentions it occasions? The pleasure of arising to a few philosophers, from seeing, a few times in their lives, the threads of light untwisted and separated by the Newtonian Prism into seven colours, can it be compared with the ease and comfort every man living might feel seven times a day, by discharging freely the wind from his bowels? Especially if it be converted into perfume; for the pleasures of one sense being little inferior to those of another, instead of pleasing the sight, he might delight in the smell of those about him, and make numbers happy, which to a benevolent mind must afford infinite satisfaction. And surely, such a liberty of expressing one's SCENT-I-MENTS, and pleasing one another, is of infinitely more importance to human happiness than the liberty of the press, or of abusing one another, which the English are so ready to fight and die for.

In short, this invention, if completed, would be, as Bacon expresses it, bringing philosophy home to men's business and bosoms. And I cannot but conclude, that in comparison therewith for universal and continual utility, the science of the philosophers aforemention'd, even with the addition, gentlemen, of your "figure quelconque," and the figures inscribed in it, are, all together, scarcely worth a FART-HING.

Life is like a box of chocolates, full of nuts and gooey sinners. Ben Franklin was a nut. Thank God. As for his turpentine pill, all I can say is, "Give 'em hell, Ben, and God bless America!" (41–accessed August 30, 2002)

## AWE SHUCKS

Leorah (pronounced "Lee'ora" ) Haley was the meanest, sweetest woman you could ever meet. Sweet and mean—sounds oxymoronic, doesn't it? For sure my Grandma Haley was oxy (heavyset), but she wasn't a moron. Smartest woman I ever knew. Grandma knew when to hold your hand and when to put her foot down. It just seemed that when she held poor old Gramps's hand, she put her foot down on his neck a lot.

Leorah weighed at least twice as much as Gramps did; she was big boned and rotund. One of my little cousins once said she liked to sleep with Grandma Haley on cold nights because she was so nice and fluffy.

My youngest brother, Tony, was still a toddler at the time. My other brother, Don, and I were just old enough to experiment with some things we probably shouldn't have. Sometimes we sneaked into a crib in the barn and smoked dry corn silks rolled in shucks. We smoked grapevines, too. But they blistered our lips. I once cut what I thought was a grapevine that turned out to be a stem of poison ivy and lit it. Corn silks didn't have such everlasting side effects. Them ivy blisters confounded Grandma and drove me nuts for a long time. I remember plain as day her looking close-up cross-eyed at my lips and tongue and saying, "I'll swear this looks just like poison ivy. You ain't been in any, have you?"

It wasn't really an outright lie I told her when I said, "In my mouth?"

That was the only lie I ever told Grandma. Funny, isn't it? How malignant lies get. You tell one . . . and another just pops out.

The Lord made me pay for that little lie to Grandma with a couple weeks of agony. My scratching my tongue on my teeth got to her, too. "Would you quit doin' that. It looks awful," she said.

"But it itches."

"I don't' care," she said and huffed. "You keep it up, you're fixin' ta git slapped."

I did learn a wonderful lesson from that precious old woman. She told me once, "Son. If you tell the truth, you don't have to remember what you said." I've tried to live by that philosophy, which I've come to call Leorah's Law.

You get my age, a lot of things don't work as well as they once did. It seems that by the time I get to where I'm going anymore, I can't remember why I went there, so I have to tell the truth. Anyway, back to the story.

My exposure to corn silk was a rather enjoyable affair, as I recall. Hidden inside that crib in the barn, my other brother, Don, and I giggled and played "grown-ups."

Gramps raised and kept lots of corn and stored it in the barn to feed his old mule, Kate. Ah, old Kate. Boy, that four-legged demon of a mule brings back memories. Gramps used Kate not only to plow with (when and only when she was in the mood) but also to pull his slide (a box made from barn lumber with sled runners). It seldom snows in East Texas. The runners were sand runners. Tony rode, while me and Don walked alongside the slide and gathered pine knots. The mature piney woods of East Texas was full of pine knots back then. Grandma used the knots to start fire with in her fireplace and in an old potbelly stove she had in her quilting room. That pine-knot scent still flags a pleasant memory now and then, especially if my wife pours pine oil in our privy. Oh, by the way, I found an old formula in a folk medicine book that told how to make a tonic for lung trouble by adding pine knot sawdust to whiskey and apple bark and molasses.

Anyway, Grandpa Haley had this problem. It seemed that about every hour or so, he disappeared behind a tree and stood with his back to us. Old men sure seemed to tinkle a lot back then.

We weren't too far from the house one day gathering pine knots when Grandma yelled to tell us that lunch was ready. Her voice carried like a bullhorn plumb across Bear Bottom. Gramps tied the mule's reins securely to a tree, and we all went to the house in a hurry; for it wasn't nice to dally around when Grandma called. Gramps stopped once to tinkle on the way home and again beside the house before going in.

Leorah was a wonderful cook. She could fix wild rabbit stew that was out of this world. I can still hear the broken hiss of that old pressure cooker bumping on the stove. By the way, wild rabbit back then was us poor folk's other white meat. Don and I used to trap rabbits in box traps Gramps showed us how to make.

After a scrumptious meal of rabbit dumplings, twice on the way back to the slide that day we detoured to check some rabbit traps. When we finally made it back to the slide where the mule was tied, we all stood in shock. That danged mule had twisted herself up in the traces and backed over a ten-foot drop off at the edge of a creek. She hanged herself good and proper—a fitting conclusion to that old outlaw's reign of terror. My brother and I had lots of corn silk to smoke after that.

Aside from the pleasure of rolling our own with no one knowing it, corn silk was used in earlier times as a medicine. That very night Grandma wadded up a fistful of the dried silks and dropped them in a small stewer of boiling water (a "stewer" is what she called a small pan with a handle that you cook with). She let that corn silk mixture steep and cool then strained the liquid through thin muslin. I don't recall ever having taken or even tasting the brew myself, but I can still smell the sweet, tamale-stench odor it left in her kitchen. Grandma had noticed Gramps tinkling a lot and made it for him. It seemed to help.

I never questioned her old corn silk brew remedy until I went to pharmacy school. To my surprise, she wasn't as far off her rocker as I at first thought. Corn silk contains tannins, which are known to have astringent effects, and cryptoxanthins, which have a vitamin-based, alterative effects on the body.

Grandma was mean to Gramps sometimes, but she loved the wiry little man, and he loved her. One cool evening in October, I remember her jumping on Gramps for something, what I can't recall—drinking a little too much, maybe—but she was unusually cruel in her accusations that night. A friend of Gramps, Tubb Wolcott, came over, and as they sat on the porch sipping moonshine and watching the peanuts grow in the field beside the house, old Tubb said, "Oscar, why do you let that damned woman run you over like that?"

Gramps took a sip from the jug. A smile that exposed a bumpy tongue and pearly pink gums bloomed on his face as he drawled, "Tubbs, old son, you ever git lucky and find yourself a good woman like Leorah, you'll learn that the benefits at private times greatly outweigh the knuckle bumps on your head. Hell, most of the time she's got good reason for what she does." Gramps sipped again and sighed to the pleasure of the brew. The wonderful silence of just sitting, relaxing, and enjoying the late of the day set in while he rolled himself a smoke of Duke's Mixture, licked, smacked, and lit it. The sweet smell of that old tobacco warmed my heart as I sat there on the porch steps near his feet. He sighed at length again and said, "Besides, Tubb, if you've roped a pissed-off mountain lion, you'll learn that you're better off donatin' *that* rope." (11–p. 69)

## HAVE A REAL DRINK, SON

His name was Orville T. Barfield. Orville had just gotten up from a restless night's sleep and was meandering along the boardwalk toward Hell's Half Acre, Fort Worth's notorious saloon section. It was quiet here now, too early for the rowdies. A mockingbird sang, "You're pretty, you're pretty," from a nearby scrub oak tree. Orville paused a moment centered in the entrance of the Trailway Saloon, then stepped through the batwings hoping to find his friend Pete Offutt inside.

"Mornin,' Orville," Pete greeted from behind the bar.

"Mornin,' Pete. Got any coffee?"

Pete picked up a pot from the top of a pot-bellied stove and swirled it. "Looks like it's all gone. Make you a fresh pot if I had anymore coffee. How about a sarsaparilla, instead?"

"Sarsaparilla'll be fine."

"You look down in the mouth, Orv. What's wrong?"

"Oh, nuthin'. Couldn't sleeps, all."

As Orville sipped his sarsaparilla, the thump of heavy boot heels and the jingle of spurs on the boardwalk outside caught his attention. He turned just as five trail-worn men entered. The man in the lead was a burly fellow with a long handlebar mustache, bushy brows, and beady eyes that moved about, deep inside of which there appeared to be movement, eyes that caught the morning light just right and reflected it like little mirrors in a glow of meanness. The man sauntered to the bar and hiked a boot on the rail. "Whiskey," he said with authority.

Orville took his sarsaparilla in hand and turned to head for a door that led to a back room, a kitchen dining area where Pete and the other employees fixed meals and ate out of view of the customers. He hadn't taken two steps to leave before a voice so deep it vibrated said, "What'sa matter, you little weasel? You too damned good to drink with the likes of us?"

Orville froze with his back to the man.

"What'ya got there?" The man said and grabbed Orville's arm, turned him, yanked that glass of sarsaparilla from his hand, and sniffed it. "What kind of pissy-assed drink is this? Barkeep, bring this boy a real drink."

Orville's heart began to race. The other four men were leaning over the bar grinning and nudging each other. These were hard-looking men, men Orville wanted no part of. Unsure of what to say, he just stood there straight-faced and blinking his eyes. Pete the barkeep placed a bottle and six empty jiggers on the bar, one before each man, then slowly slid one toward Orville. Pete's face was totally devoid of expression.

"Drink up," the burly man said.

"I'm just minding my own business, mister," Orville replied, "No disrespect, sir, but I don't drink."

The man eased back his coat and placed his hand on the biggest pistol Orville had ever seen. The man narrowed his brows and barked, "I said, drink."

The other men leaned over the bar to better see and once again elbowed one another.

The only other time Orville had tasted whiskey it made him sick. But he'd rather be sick than die. He took the jigger delicately between a thumb and finger and deadpan tossed it. The vile brew made it halfway down before it changed its mind. His tongue and throat burned like he'd swallowed a glass of jalapeño pepper juice. His vision blurred. He tried hard to swallow again and was on the brink of unfathomable discomfort when the man said, "That ain't so bad now, is it?" and grinned and flung a proud look toward the others.

Orville's stomach chose that instant to draw up in a knot; his back became manfully erect, and he expelled a gurgling stream that splattered on the floor at the men's feet. Every face in the house grimaced. As if an invisible cloud had passed down the bar, each man in sequence bolted toward the door. The mean man's face, the one with the penetrating eyes who started all this, had a pale cast to it. Those powerful pupils quickly lost their luster and became surrounded by a puny squint. He let out a quick groan that started low and got higher in pitch as his stomach jerked. He had his palm on his belt buckle when he, too, stormed out the door.

Orville stared across the now-vacant room. His lips were sticky and his tongue felt pasty as he wiped the back of a hand across his face and moved his tongue about. To the bitter taste of bile, he shook his head, a gentle move that sent a quiver up his spine. He stood there a moment before taking another sip of his sarsaparilla, which, by the way, helped settle his stomach.

This story fits the typical image of we think about sarsaparilla. But was it really served in old western saloons to dudes and greenhorns, or was its association to cowboys contrived by Hollywood?

Sarsaparilla beers have been around since medieval times. In nineteenth-century Europe, the lack of sanitation, as well as drinking water collected from rains and stored for long periods or from shallow wells infested with bloated frogs or rotting rats, often made children sick.

Legend has it that a monk in Belgium studied why rich people lived longer than poor folks and found that the well-to-do drank more beer and wine than water. The tradition of monastic beer brewing to bring cheaper beer to the poor continues to this day in that country. It became apparent from this study that low alcohol content was an important necessity if these drinks were to be consumed by children. Beers were sought that contained less than 2 percent alcohol. These low concentrations acted purely as preservatives to make the drinks safer longer.

"Small beers," as they were referred to, unlike regular beers and ales made from infusions of malt by fermentation, were made more like teas by boiling roots and herbs to kill the bacteria, then cooled and minimally fermented with yeast. Honey, molasses, and cane sugar were used as sweeteners.

Fermentation produced not only the necessary alcohol but also a bubbly effervescence. Saponins in sarsaparilla gave the drink a foamy head and a characteristic bitterroot flavor. These crude, weak beers were consumed very early in the fermentation process while still sweet and flavored with the herbs and natural sugars used.

The first Americans to settle on the East Coast built houses, and towns—and breweries. Even in these civilized surroundings, frontiersmen did things for themselves: bread making, weaving and sewing their own clothes, and brewing their own regular beers, ales for adults and small beers for their children. Colonists prepared their children's beers from naturally flavored roots like sarsaparilla and sassafras, birch bark, burdock root, vanilla beans, prickly ash bark, dandelion, cinnamon, ginger, and numerous other plants. There were as many pioneer recipes for home made root beers as there were for apple pie. The most popular with the children were sarsaparilla, birch bark, ginger, and sassafras.

An inventive pharmacist named Charles Hires popularized small beers at the Philadelphia Centennial Exhibition in 1876 by introducing the first commercially available root beer to the public. Hires Herb Tea extract produced a product similar to the sarsaparilla beers made at home yet was much easier to prepare. In addition to sarsaparilla and sassafras, his concoction contained juniper, spikenard, wintergreen, vanilla beans, ginger, hops, dog grass, and licorice. His next logical step was to produce a finished, ready-to-drink bottled product. In 1893, under his guidance, the Crystal Bottling Company began bottling sarsaparilla and distributing it. Hires naturally promoted his drinks as healthful and sold them through apothecary outlets. The sassafras in Hire's Extract came from the root of a tree indigenous to the south. Safrole, a volatile oil in sassafras root, was determined by the Food and Drug Administration (FDA) to have carcinogenic properties and was later outlawed.

Frontiersmen used sarsaparilla more for its curative qualities than for making beverages. Medicinal sarsaparilla was and still is listed in many official compendiums: in the tenth revision of *The Pharmacopoeia of the United States*, in *Remington's Pharmaceutical Sciences*, and in the modern *Natural Medicines/Comprehensive Database.*

The drug's medicinal use dates back to the early sixteenth century. The Chinese called it *tu fu ling* and used it as a treatment for venereal disease and as an aphrodisiac. The medicinal sarsaparilla preparations consumed by American cowboys were said to make them more virile and helped ward off the nasty infections they acquired after going to brothels. Sarsaparilla root stimulated the healthy flow of urine to cleanse the urinary tract. The remedies were also taken to relieve aching backs and the sore butt bones (arthritis and rheumatism) pursuant to spending long periods in the saddle or sitting for hours on a hard buckboard seat.

The saponin glycosides in sarsaparilla have binding actions with toxins in the gut and were used to treat poisonings due to mercury and silver and other heavy metals. Powdered and prepared in ointments, the root was used for psoriasis and other skin diseases. Combined into compounds containing iron, along with natural tonics like yellow dock and stillingia, and the alterative mandrake root (a natural laxative), the remedies were sold to help the weak get stronger. Iron added to these compounds had as much to do with the remedy's success as did the sarsaparilla. Iron deficiency in women and children is still a problem today.

Mexico and Central America were primary sources of the raw product. The name *Zarza para illa* was Spanish, meaning a "small, twisting vine." Zarzaparilla was prepared from the orange-hued roots of the *Smilax linné* plant (family Liliaceae). The applicable parts being the root, its active ingredients were quercetin and phytosterols, all of which had diuretic (increased urine flow and kidney function), diaphoretic (made you sweat out toxins), expectorant (loosened and thinned phlegm in the upper respiratory tract), and laxative action. These compounds stimulated the flow of digestive juices and helped improve appetite and digestion. A typical dose of medicinal sarsaparilla was one to four grams of the dried and pulverized root, or one cup of a tea prepared by steeping a teaspoonful of the powder in boiling water for five to ten minutes, straining and taking. An alcoholic extract prepared by mixing one part powdered root with one part whiskey was dosed at one to three teaspoonfuls three times a day.

The sarsaparilla compounds that came west on pack trains, freight wagons, and later by railway were mostly packaged or prepared in the east. Nineteenth-century manufacturers produced calendars, almanacs, and elaborate sales cards for retailers to pass out at churches and other gatherings. The two most successful distributors during the period hailed from Lowell, Massachusetts: Dr. J. C. Ayer and Co. and C. I. Hood & Co., Apothecaries. Their sales cards displayed intricate lithographic pictures, the backs of which contained sales pitches aimed mostly at women and children.

The image of sarsaparilla as a low-alcohol beverage commonly sold in western saloons to dudes and greenhorns was due in part to a man named Hubert Hansen who, in 1935, earned a loyal following among Hollywood movie studio employees that favored a drink he produced. Hansen's Sarsaparilla was how the drink got its humble beginnings in wide-screen western saloons and became a movie star on its own. True, an occasional local brew master may have offered his own version of a small beer at local bars, but as a common drink, sarsaparilla, or low- or no-alcohol root beer, was sold less in rowdy saloons than at soda fountains. As a medicine mostly druggists at apothecaries sold it.

The name *sarsaparilla* has become synonymous with all root beers, and since there are so many inexpensive and more effective products on the market, medicinal sarsaparilla is seldom if ever used. Modern root beers contain no true sarsaparilla or sassafras root. Artificial oils that mimic their tastes have taken their places.

## A BIZARRE BRASSIERE

The Guernsey has long been the best of the milk-producing cows. It wasn't uncommon for the old females to produce as much as thirteen gallons of milk a day. The Guernsey with the largest udder ever recorded was named Lucy and lived in North Carolina. Her udder measured twelve feet. Imagine dragging that across the cactus- and grass-burr-strewn pastures of the American west. It's hard to imagine a cow with an udder capable of holding six gallons of milk, which isn't all that uncommon even today.

The Lohmann Brothers Dairy at Nederland, Texas, was famous for its milk cows. Back then all milking was done by hand. The Lohmann Brothers babied their cows with low lights and plush, clean barns. They measured an animal's feed in precise amounts based on the number of gallons of milk they produced per day. The cows with the largest udders stayed inside, mostly. The ones that were allowed to browse in the pastures were harnessed with huge brassieres fashioned from burlap bags to help transfer the udder's weight more to the backbone—a cross-your-heart, m-o-o-ving experience, which was "udderly" comforting, I'm sure.

Milk was in earlier times thought to have healing properties. It still is Mother Nature's perfect food. When you remember that God designed cow's milk to make a calf gain two hundred pounds in six months, you realize the vitamin and nutritional properties milk

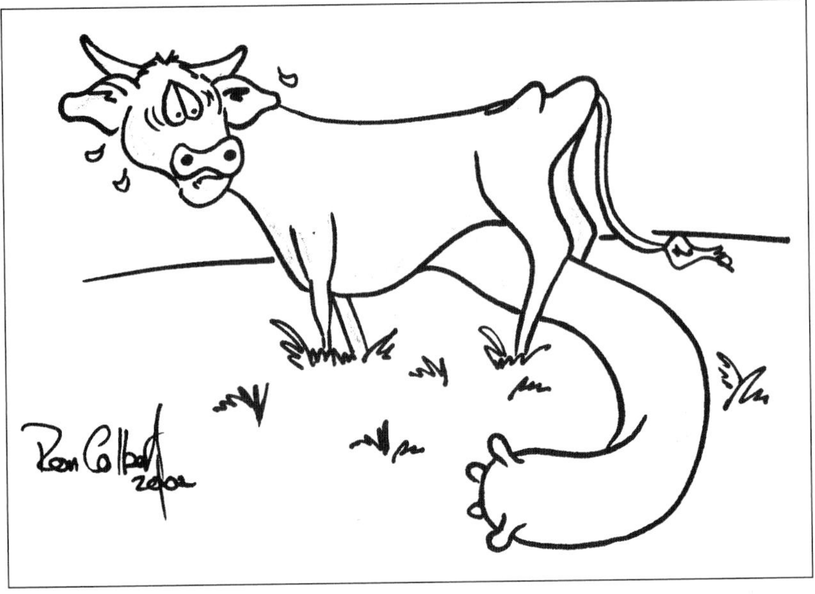

offers. Most of milk's healing properties in frontier times had more to do with its vitamin and nutritional content than anything. Raw milk's stomach-soothing qualities may have been due to the fatty liquid's high calcium amounts, that or the bacteria it contained that helped restore the normal flora of bacteria to the bowel. What with all the purgatives pioneers took back then, it's no wonder they needed that replaced.

The first milk produced by mammals after birth contains colostrums, a thin, yellow fluid secreted from the breasts or udders. Colostrums contain immunoglobulins and antibodies found in the mother's blood—nature's own way of passing a mother's immunity on to her offspring. Breastfeeding is still the best thing a mother can do for her child, especially during its first few weeks.

Like the potato, milk's medicinal value lies solely with its dietary benefits. But in a time when vitamins were unheard of and food was scarce, those vitamins did have healing properties.

The "Got milk?" ads of today continue to reinforce our passion for the nectar of the teat. Our waistlines? Well, they directly reflect the nutritious value milk affords. Two hundred pounds in six months? No wonder my pants are tight. And I thought it was the cookies. (30–accessed August 13, 2002)

## AN APRON FULL OF GUT

The annals of medical history are full of amazing, even astounding facts. This story, a true anecdote that lies somewhere between miracle and marvel, was fictionally enhanced to exemplify just how brutal life was in the days of old.

"How you feelin,' Homer?"

"Some better. I'll be fine. Just let me rest. Should be as good as new by tomorrow."

Evyleen Bradbury straightened her back after feeling of her husband's forehead. He'd been down three days now with high fever and a horrible backache. She'd just given him another dose of anodyne bitters Dr. Traweek had left here on his visit two days before. Homer's color was better. Evyleen glanced toward the kitchen when the back door screen banged. "I gotta go milk," she said to Homer, then she yelled toward the door. "Leroy, you stay in here and watch your papa till I git back. You hear me?"

"Yes, ma'am," the eight-year-old replied.

Homer rose to an elbow, "Honey, that young Jersey ain't as tame as old Bessie was. You better wait and let me do the milking. Won't hurt to let her go another day. Why don't you just let the calf have her again till I feel better? "

"You stay put. I been kicked by a cow before," she said.

"It ain't her feet I'm worried about," Homer replied as he went through the motions of getting up.

"Stay put," Evyleen insisted. "She acts up too much, I'll just turn her out. "

Homer eased back down, sighed to the pain his movement had caused, and closed his eyes. Evyleen walked to him and patted him on the shoulder. "I'll be all right. You rest now, you hear me?" She tied on an apron, put a little water in a milk bucket to wash the cows' teats, and headed for the barn. The Jersey was already in position with her head at the feed trough, so Evyleen got her stool, placed it on the ground beside the cow, and dipped several scoops of mixed oats and corn into the trough. The Jersey squared off and hooked its curved horns menacingly, left then right. As the animal stared, it licked its lips and then ran its tongue up one nostril and then the other.

"Back off, you heifer."

The cow stood her ground but glanced at the fresh feed. That was when Evyleen made the mistake of turning her back to pick up the stool and bucket. The big Jersey was on her before she realized. Evyleen turned but didn't have time to even yell before one quick swoop of a sharp horn hit her in the side. Pain like she'd been stabbed with a white-hot branding iron shot through her stomach. It took a moment to realize what had happened. It was the steam of her own entrails rising into her face that made her realize she'd been gored wide open from one side of the belly to the other. The cow, as if nothing had happened, walked to the trough and began to feed.

Evyleen went slowly to her knees as her own shiny entrails wormed and ran warm down her thighs and onto the ground. She came to sit on her heels. Nausea loomed. Amazingly, there was very little blood—just a glob of what reminded her of huge chicken guts gaining in mass in the dirt between her knees. She looked to the cow, toward the house, back down. What the hell to do now? The next thing she knew, she was scooping up her own guts into her apron. That done, she held the corners of the cloth in one hand and pushed to stand with the other. It amazed her how heavy her entrails were and how cold the air felt just now. Dizziness made her wobble; a faint lingered.

"Leeeeroy?" she screamed. The back screen door clapped twice and in an instant the child ran to her. She could see Homer walking stiffly down the steps to come to her aid.

"Oh, my God," Homer swore when he reached her. His eyes were wide, and he wasn't moving slow no more. "Leroy," he yelled. "Git on the mule and go git Doc Traweek. Hurry!"

Homer helped her inside and immediately began throwing back covers on the bed. Evyleen walked stiffly to the bedside and took a seat. "I might better sit in a chair till Doc gits here. Don't think I kin lie down like this."

Homer seemed indecisive. His face was pale as a sheet as he fidgeted trying to decide what to do. His hand felt firm in her armpit as he helped her to her favorite old rocker beside the fireplace. She knew he needed something to do, so she said, "Stoke up the fire, would ya? I'm cold." Homer hurried out to do just that.

She wasn't sure whether she passed out or not, but everything was suspended in a haze for the next hour or so. She couldn't stop her legs from shaking. Once while she sat there waiting for the doctor, her hand cramped and she almost lost her grip on her apron. Homer reached as if to help but withdrew when she grabbed the corners with the other hand and repositioned the bloody wad in her lap. Rocking ever so slightly, she sat there feeling the warmth of her own blood run into other private places. It seemed forever before heavy boots thumped on the porch floor and the screen door banged.

She recognized Dr. Traweek's tenor voice when he said, "Jeesus Christ!" and hurried to her side.

Everything that happened next occurred in dreamy state. They placed her on the dining table, on her side, while the doctor examined her entrails. He gave her several droppers full of a bitter-tasting liquid, and soon the pain stopped. "Boil me a big pan of water," Doc instructed Homer. "Git me some wet rags. We gotta keep these moist. Put two teaspoonfuls of salt in the pan, boil it good, then set it on the porch to cool, and fix another one. Put the same amount of salt in the second pan, along with twenty drops of this."

"What is this stuff, Doc?" Homer asked as he held the tiny dropper bottle to the light.

Doctor Traweek spoke as he worked. "Silver nitrate. I'm hoping it'll keep the infection down. We gotta wash all the dirt and manure off these entrails before I can put them back in. But first, this bowel has got to be stitched."

It took Dr. Traweek half the night to clean all the manure and grit off, gently place those entrails back inside, and stitch Evyleen up. It was a miracle she lived to milk again, but she did.

Albert Carroll Traweek was a physician who practiced in Motley County, Texas, for over sixty-two years. He was born in Comanche on December 1, 1875, and lived to be a ripe old eighty-four. The good doctor was one of Texas' first "saddlebag" physicians. Dr. Traweek later became a horse-and-buggy doctor, took to a motorcycle as time progressed, and finally bought the first automobile in Motley County. As for the woman the milk cow gored, very little is known; even her name has been fictionalized here to tell her and Dr. Traweek's story.

The salt solution the good doctor supposedly prepared in this anecdote, two teaspoonfuls to a gallon of sterile water, is essentially normal saline, the same solution given intravenously today to restore fluid volume. Dr. Traweek had to have used a balanced solution of some kind to wash off the lady's entrails, for it is well known that plain water is hypo-osmotic and if applied to entrails can cause a fatal electrolyte imbalance. Silver nitrate is still used as an antibiotic. The American Academy of Pediatrics endorses to this day placing two drops of a 1 percent solution in newborn babies' eyes to prevent gonorrheal blindness. (10; 32–accessed August 12, 2002)

## CUFF'S BLUFF: "BY GAWD, HE'S A GIRL!"

Hands behind back, rocking from heel to toe, Colonel Orlando Poe stood before a window in his office. The Rebels were up to something, he just knew it. Things were much too quiet. "We've got to get someone in there. Who do we have?" he said as he turned at the waist to face Captain Lance Albright, his second in command.

"No one I can think of, except maybe Frank Thompson."

The colonel faced the window again. "What we need is a black man to get in there among them confederate slaves and find out what the hell is going on." He then turned toward his desk. The chair vibrated as he pulled it back. "Get Thompson for me, Captain, I've got an idea that just might work."

Less than an hour later, the colonel pushed back his chair, and with his elbows on the desk, he steepled his fingers and touched them to his lips. "Whad'ya you think, Frank?"

Frank Thompson, a beardless soldier, small in stature and with a voice as high-pitched as a woman's, sat now staring out the window. His brows were narrowed in study. He broke his trance to take a small bottle from the desktop. Turning it up to saturate a rag, he dabbed it to the back of his hand. "I think it just might work. Might need to dilute it a little more. You know this stuff is darned near permanent? "

The colonel laughed. "Yeah, but if you can pull it off, it will be worth it," and he and stood. "Get ready and I'll arrange your transport to the front lines." The colonel then paused and relaxed his face and stuck out his hand. Thompson took it and shook, limply. "You be careful, Frank, you hear me? Don't take any chances. Just meander in there among them darkies and listen. Then come straight back after dark. And thanks again. Your country will owe you for this one."

And her country did owe her, a lot more than anyone realizes. Yes, I said "her." The real Frank Thompson was a female, an incognito woman, serving a full stretch in the Union Army in 1862. And that wasn't the only mission she went on as a man and as a spy for Colonel Poe and the Union Army. Frank Thompson's real name was Sarah Emma Edmundson. (I found *Edmundson* spelled *Edmondson* and *Edmonds* in several different research resources.)

Many of the soldiers she served with never knew she was a woman until an army reunion in 1884 where she shocked them by showing up as her true self—Sarah Emma Evelyn Edmundson Seelye (1841–1898), alias Frank Thompson—nurse, mother of five, spy, Secret Service agent, woman impersonator, deserter, the first woman member of the Grand Army of the Republic, *and* one of the first publisher's agents in the midwestern United States.

Canadian born, Sarah Edmundson, at the age of seventeen and dressed as a man, in 1839 ran away from home in New Brunswick to escape a demanding father. In 1861, she took the name Frank Thompson, and when President Abraham Lincoln pleaded for volunteers in his Union Army, she set out to enlist. She tried three times to join but didn't succeed until the fourth attempt to become a "man" in the army. With her being of such small stature, she, or rather he, became a nurse, serving as a dispatch carrier until she (he) became a spy for the army. At one time she, under the ruse of a "he," pretended to be a "she," which he really was, and wandered through Confederate camps as Bridget O'Shea, an Irish peddler who sold possibles—matches, thread, writing paper, soap, and other articles—to Rebel soldiers. As she went about her job, she kept a keen ear for information about troop movement and battle strategy. She once returned with information that the Rebels were not as strong a force as they appeared and that the cannons they displayed on a hill overlooking a wide expanse of the Union's approach were dummies made from logs and painted black with pitch tar.

The story of why she deserted the army is recorded two ways. One source says she left because she and a soldier she was in love with broke up. Another historical researcher says she deserted because she feared being found out when she went to the hospital to be treated for a severe case of ague (malaria).

Later, after having heard that Frank Thompson's name had appeared on the deserters list, she rejoined the army as a female nurse in Washington, where she worked until the war ended. Before that she sold for a publishing house and represented herself with her own book, *Nurse and Spy in the Union Army*, a scandalous fictional account of her life as a spy, which she got published in 1865 and sold well over 150,000 copies, all the profits of which she donated to the war cause.

Some of her many ruses were Frank Thompson, a Union soldier; Cuff, a black male spy (depicted at the beginning of this story in which she painted herself with silver nitrate to make her skin black); Bridget O'Shea, the traveling Irish peddler; and Charles

Mayberry, a man who rousted out informers on the Union Army in Tennessee.

She wasn't a born-again virgin who didn't like men, either. Sarah returned to Canada after the war, married Linus Seelye, came back to the States, and gave birth to a total of five or three, depending on the historian, children, all but one of whom died in infancy.

Sarah, encouraged by her family, was finally cleared of her deserter status. In 1884, during a March 28 convening of the House of Representatives, a bill was passed that validated her claims for a government pension.

Sarah Emma Evelyn Edmundson Seelye died where she lived in La Porte, Texas, on September 5, 1898. She lies interred to this day in Houston, at the Washington Cemetery.

During the Civil War, many women tried to serve in the army as men; nearly four hundred have been recorded, but no one knows exactly how many did it and were never discovered. If those women had been anything like Sarah Seeley, and General Armstrong Custer had had four hundred of them with him at the Little Big Horn or, better yet, if he'd had four hundred of my Grandma Leorah Haley's with him, there wouldn't have been any Indians left, period.

I can't for the life of me imagine anyone painting themselves with silver nitrate. Every time I try to conjure up an image of how soot-black and maybe mottled and blistered Sarah's skin must have looked, my Aunt Willa Dean's face (with that gentian violet coming out of her nose) pops into my mind. But, Sarah did it—bigger than life. This nation owes a lot to its women, doesn't it? (33–August 12, 2002)

## THERE'S A TEAR IN MY BEER, DEAR

They were somewhere outside Canton, Ohio, when the man beside her ran a hand up Billie Jean's dress. "Dammit, quit—you're drunk," she snapped.

She wrestled with him, all the while digging her heels into the floorboard. But he had a firm grip on the inside of her thigh. God, he was drunk-man strong. She grabbed his wrist and tore his hold loose, placed both of her hands on his shoulders, and pushed him into the corner of the backseat. "Quit it, I said. You'll git my new dress all wrinkled."

The man's smile died by degrees as he flopped back. The way the passing streetlights came through the tinted windows made it look like she was seeing him in an old black-and-white movie. She glanced away and bit her bottom lip when he fumbled around in his suit pocket and palmed a handful of pills, which he stared at a moment before throwing them into his mouth. Trying desperately to swallow, he coughed and took a swig from a half-full fifth of whiskey he had stashed beside him. He took another drink, and yet another.

"Honey, don't git stoned again, please?" Billie Jean pleaded.

He waved her off, slid even farther down in the seat, and slouched there staring out the window. Just as the limousine sped into the bright lights of a small business community, she heard him singing, softly, ". . . and melt your c-o-o-ld c-o-o-ld heart."

"Henry, when does the show start?" Billie Jean asked.

The driver lowered the partition window a little more and centered his eyes in the rearview mirror. "There's plenty-a time. Don't worry. We'll make it. Just keep him sober if you can."

Billie Jean cast a quick glance into the shadows beside her. Hank's eyes were shut now, his head was tilted back, and his mouth was open a little. "Honey, you OK?" She asked.

He grunted and pulled his hat down over his eyes. "I'm fine. Le've me alone."

Billie Jean left her husband alone that night, but she shouldn't have. He went to sleep in the backseat of that limousine and never woke up. He fulfilled the lifelong prophecy of a song he wrote but didn't get to sing in Canton, Ohio, that night, a song titled "I'll Never Git Out of This World Alive." His death was caused by a suspected overdose of alcohol and chloral and/or opium. Some say the drugs combined with alcohol were what killed him; some say the combination precipitated a fatal heart attack.

In 1954, two songs Billie Jean's husband recorded, "Why Don't You Love Me?" and "Long Gone Lonesome Blues," made it to the top of the country music charts.

His son, Hank Williams Jr., became a recording artist, too. A duo, which Junior dubbed and recorded with his deceased father, was recently a huge hit. That song is titled "There's a Tear in My Beer."

The famous Hank Williams Sr. toured the country many times before he died. His body rests today in the Oakwood Annex Cemetery in Montgomery, Alabama.

## RATS!

A Yankee once said to me and laughed, "Hey, are you one of them Texas guys that eats possum and Irish taters? I hear you folks eat a lot of them big rats down here."

I squinted through a frown. Nothing rankles me more than having someone stab at my southern heritage. A man from Kansas, whom I did like, once joked, "I love it the way you Texans criticize someone, then immediately feel sorry for it, and apologize for their rudeness."

It took a moment for that one to sink in.

At a local pharmacy recently, after the cashier checked them out, two women walked away talking. One leaned to the other and said, "If one more person says 'Have a nice day,' I think I'll vomit. I can't wait to get back to the Bronx."

I thought, "I can't wait for you to get back there, either, lady."

Anyway, anyone with country savvy knows you don't eat possum with Irish potatoes; you eat them with sweet taters. I'm afraid, though, that New Yorker might have me on the rat part. Possums are the blonds of the varmint world, and I think they really are members of the rat family. There isn't much sport in hunting them. Poor folks only eat them when there isn't anything else. But there is one thing besides a dog we southerners won't eat (if we know it), and that's a rat. Just writing about them gives me the willies.

> The houses were filled with dead bodies . . . neither age nor sex was exempt; slaves and plebeians were suddenly taken off amidst the lamentations of their wives and children, who, while they assisted the sick and mourned the dead, were seized with the disease and, perishing, were burned on the same funeral pyre.

And so goes the account of the bubonic plague that struck Imperial Rome, and which throughout frontier times occurred over and again. And yep, I had to look *plebian* up, too. It means "crude or course in the manner of style," as in one of the "common" people.

Black Death, or the bubonic plague, as it's called, was caused by a bacillus, a bacteria transmitted by rat fleas. A patient contracting the disease presented with tumors in the groin and in the armpits, some as large as horse apples, and afterward, purple areas developed on the skin like huge black bruises that eventually consumed the body. Black Death wreaked havoc on Asian immigrants.

Frontiersmen, particularly those residing in shipping areas like Galveston and New Orleans, were ignorant of bacteriology and the source of the disease. Black Death's association with rats was so obvious that no one could see it at first.

P. L. Simond of Spain conceived the theory that fleas from rats caused the plague. Every year afterward confirmed the theory. An outbreak in Bombay showed that guinea pigs harbored rat fleas, and dead rats were found everywhere. A simple experiment proved the theory. Caged rats were hung at different heights from the floor where fleas exposed to dead and infected animals were placed. The healthy rats that dangled within the four-inch jump span of the fleas contracted the disease and died. The fortunate ones were those higher above the floor. You don't reckon that's why my wife climbs in a chair when she sees a rat, do you? And I thought she was just scared.

Any rat can harbor the plague. The major culprit, though, is the long-tailed, blackish *Mus rattus*, commonly called the "wharf rat." *Mus norwegicus*, the reddish-gray, shorter-tailed rat, better known as the "field rat," avoids humans. Hence, the primary areas stricken with the plague were slums and shipping areas where old *Mus rattus* thrived on human food. Ships arriving in American ports were infested with rats from abroad. Many of the vessels that docked in Port Galveston during frontier days were de-ratted and disinfected by battening down the hatches and burning sulfur in large metal pots. Dr. Victor Heiser, in his book *An American Doctor's Odyssey*, relates an occasion where a ship from the Philippines was disinfected using these crude sulfur bombs. Within minutes of setting the sulfur afire, Chinese stowaways began coming out of the woodwork. Dr. Heiser reported, "In front of our astonished eyes, forty coughing coolies, one after another, emerged with streaming eyes through a thick veil of billowing yellow smoke."

A plague-stricken rat, like a person, develops a fever and septicemia. He becomes sluggish and fears nothing. When he dies, the fleas abandon him and seek shelter in wood cracks and crevices; these sneaky little critters can live up two months. In lieu of a live rat, they seek out humans, squirrels, and even marmots. Frontiersmen around rat-infested slum areas or docks went barefoot a lot and rolled up their pants legs. This afforded the fleas easy pickin's; they simply hopped aboard and began to feast.

The rats in New York, the four-legged kind, were estimated at the end of the nineteenth century to eat a penny's worth of food a day on shore and twice that aboard ships where garbage was thrown overboard.

The United States Public Health Service, in 1924, finally studied the rat problem and began "ratproofing" ships and wharfs. The British, the Dutch, and the Germans followed suit. But the French, well, they just didn't care. Their shipments from abroad were the most likely to harbor the dreaded Black Death, with New York being the primary hot spot for outbreaks for long, long time. I guess that's why there are still so many rats in New York.

I'm sorry. New Yorkers aren't rats—plebeians, maybe, but then, heck, they can't help it, bless their hearts. (36–p. 79)

## AMERICA'S FIRST "LADY" DOCTOR

The dean of the Geneva College of Medicine in upstate New York read the letter slowly, looked up, down, up again. This had to be approached with care. He didn't want his office involved in anymore scandal or ridicule. "How do you think we oughta handle this?"

His faculty associate walked to the window and stood looking out across campus. It was early. The windows were open. A cool, September breeze swirled the curtains. The "teakettle-teakettle" warble of a Carolina wren echoed from across the way.

"We can't let this happen," his associate said. "Perhaps, you could present it to the students and let them make the final decision. That would take the heat off you . . . and me, and the rest of faculty."

With his palms flat on the desk, the dean pushed back. He stood, removed a watch from his pocket, and fumbled with it. "Excellent idea. Come on."

As the dean read the letter to the class, silence fell over the lecture hall. Everyone in attendance appeared as if stricken by paralysis. Someone dropped a pencil. The dean stopped reading, looked up, and then went on. He finished and folded his spectacles, placing them carefully inside his suit pocket. Every face glared at him in a blue hue, which was cast from the high windows in the lecture hall. "We will only accede to this request," he added with authority, "by a unanimous vote of this student body."

For a moment, the ludicrousness of the situation seized the whole class. Sweeping babble and laughter followed. The dean stood there trying to hold back a smile. "Calm down. Calm down. Let's put it to the vote and be done with it." He had to raise his voice to be heard as he added, "All in favor, say 'aye.'"

His brows narrowed when every student in the room stood, and

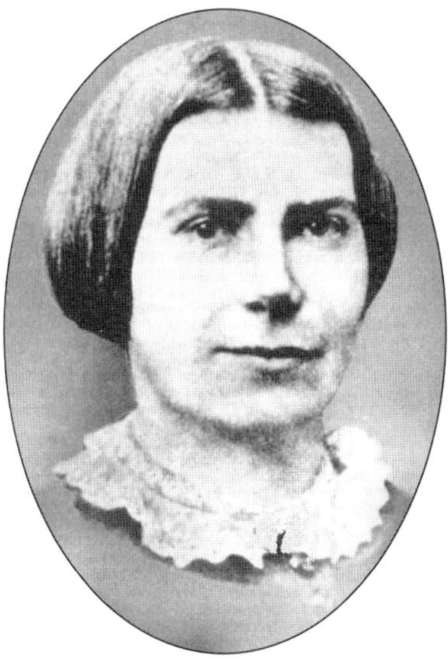

***Elizabeth Blackwell (1821–1910), first certified lady physician in America***

in a fit of jocular activity, waving handkerchiefs and tossing hats into the air, everyone called out, "Aye!" in roaring unison.

The dean glanced at the faculty that lined the left side of the lecture hall. Every instructor's face was straight, every mouth open a little.

Over a fortnight passed before on another cool morning in the fall of 1847 the dean reentered the lecture hall. A hush fell over the room as he stepped to the podium. With a trembling voice, he said, "Gentlemen. Let me introduce . . . Miss Elizabeth Blackwell." Deathlike stillness prevailed when the first woman ever accepted to attend the Geneva College of Medicine entered the room.

On October 20, 1847, Elizabeth Blackwell (1821–1910), after months of rejections, was accepted to the Geneva Medical College. But her acceptance was the result of backfire in plans. The students who voted "aye" that day thought that the dean's request had been a joke.

Miss Blackwell's success was a huge victory for women, but her male classmates were anything but cooperative. They failed to document in the charts of the patients seen by her. Still, she prevailed, and she graduated at the top of her class.

During her years of tending the ill and sick, Elizabeth comforted many. One of her doctoring experiences had personal repercussions that nearly ended her career. In November 1849, while tending a child with infected eyes (probably pinkeye), she accidentally splashed contaminated water into her own face. A few days later her eye became so inflamed it was swollen shut, and the pain from it put her in bed. A fellow physician, Dr. Hippolyte Blot, treated her with compresses, leeches, ointments, and even footbaths, but nothing worked. After many days of agony, the eye had to be removed. Elizabeth practiced thereafter seeing her patients through only one eye.

Following in her footsteps, her sister, Emily Blackwell (1826–1910), was accepted as a student at the Rush Medical College in Chicago. Elizabeth tried to warn her sister of the consequences and the adversity she would face as a woman in medicine. Elizabeth's warning's came to fruition when, bowing to pressure, after a year the college rescinded Emily's admission. Emily traveled to Western Reserve Medical College in Cleveland, where in March 1854 she graduated with honors.

Elizabeth died in 1910, within a few months of her sister Emily. In that same year, there were over six thousand women physicians practicing in the United States. Today, some of our most prominent physicians are women. To that we owe an immeasurable debt to the determined efforts of frontier women the likes of Elizabeth and Emily Blackwell. Men cut off their arrogance to spite their pride sometimes, don't they?

Rebecca J. Cole, the second black woman to receive a medical degree, worked under Elizabeth Blackwell. Dr. Cole spent fifty years in medicine, was the founder of the Woman's Directory, a Philadelphia institution offering legal aid to women in medicine, and also founded the National Association of Colored Women. (38–p. 59; 37–p. 58)

## BAREFOOT AND PREGNANT—FOR A LONG, LONG TIME

Sometime in 1899, a thirteen-year-old girl squirmed beneath her first lover. Afterward she fought nausea and stomach cramps, but she never got a large tummy like most pregnant girls did. She simply hurt, hurt bad, for a long, long time. She later married but never had children.

In May 1979, that little girl (now an old woman) went to a doctor when the recurring cramps got so bad she couldn't stand it. The doctor X-rayed her abdomen and found something neither he nor she could believe. Now, at the age of eighty-three, she was pregnant. Surgery was scheduled, and—seventy years after having conceived an ectopic pregnancy, a totally calcified fetus, complete with identifiable extremities, was removed. The woman had carried that baby all that time. That's a heck of a long time to have phantom symptoms and put-down pain. It's a long time to be pregnant, too.

(This story was reported in the *Houston Chronicle*, June 3, 1979, sec. 3, p. 32, as per reference 37–p. 5.)

## WOUND SUCKING ON THE SLY

A number of old-time remedies seem outlandish today. This story enlightens with one of the first "accepted" surgical procedures known.

Robert went to his knees when the arrow entered his arm. Such pain he had never imagined. The tip had buried so firmly in bone it was all his wife, Sybillia, could do to pull it out with both hands.

Sybillia, like most frontier women, was a faithful wife, beautiful, caring, a lady of distinguished accomplishments for whom Robert had sacrificed a lot to gain the favor of.

After a few days on the trail to the next outpost, the wound got worse, much worse. Pain made it difficult for Robert to remain in the saddle. Though Sybillia had bandaged the arm with strips torn from her own pantaloons, the wound festered into a running sore. Robert nearly went out of his head with fever and wouldn't let her even look at or replace the soggy dressing and clean the wound.

Robert consulted with doctors once they reached town and was told that the only way to get the injury to heal was to remove the poison by sucking it out. None of the doctors offered to personally draw the poison out but insisted it needed to be done. Robert didn't like the idea, anyway. It would hurt too much.

That night, taking advantage of husband's pain-induced semi-coma of sleep, Sybillia fell to her knees beside him, placed her lips over the oozing hole, and sucked every bit of the puss and poison out of that arrow hole. Robert recovered fully as a result.

The medical men who suggested the treatment later wrote a textbook about hygiene and the use of this drawing method in a volume titled *Regimen Sanitatis Salernitanum.*

Wound sucking by mouth, or the use of cupping devices, was a quite common affair in the days of old. We've all heard of sucking the poison out of snakebites. The same went for puncture sores like splinters, bullet and arrow holes, and such.

This true incident in history didn't take place on America's frontier as the story leads one to believe. It happened over eight hundred years ago, in Europe. Robert was his real name; only it was Robert, Duke of Normandy, son of William the Conqueror. Sybillia was his wife, for whose sake he gave up a chance at the English throne. Robert's injury really was from an arrow, the festered hole of which Sybillia did indeed suck clean to save his life.

That book, *Regimen Sanitatis Salernitanum*, which touted the use of wound sucking, was so popular it went into over two hundred editions and was *the* compendium on medicine during Queen Elizabeth's reign. Many of early America's remedies and medicinal practices came from books that came from Europe. A cute quote from a page in the *Regimen Sanitatis Salernitanum* goes:

And scorn not Garlick, like to some that think
It only makes men wink, and drink, and stink. (40–p. 144)

This story gives a whole new meaning to "Oh, how I love thee," don't it? Anyway, after writing this piece and having read it to my wife, one night while we sat before the television watching a love story that put us both on the verge of tears, I said, "Honey, I love you enough to suck a running sore for you."

A forced smile warped her right cheek as she said, "You're such a romantic."

## SAVING GRACE

It started at the back of Grace Danforth's head and spread slowly, like someone hammering a metal rod on an anvil to make the tip flat, the pounding keeping beat with her heart. The pain got so bad that blackness crept in at the edges of her vision. She'd had bad headaches before, but nothing like this. With a straight arm, she braced herself on the nightstand. She had to get to her medicine bag. For sure, laudanum wasn't something she normally took, medicine was for use on her patients, but she simply couldn't take this pain much longer. One dropper full, then another, and still another, until the pressure inside her skull began to subside, not completely, but enough to allow her to catch her breath and stagger to the bed. Before she eased her head back onto the pillow, she took yet another dose of laudanum, placed the bottle on the nightstand, closed her eyes, and sighed. Dr. Grace Danforth died that dreary night of February 21, 1895.

Grace Danforth (1849–1895) was an accomplished Texas physician. She studied medicine at the Women's Medical Center in Chicago and did her internship at the Chicago Hospital for Women and Children. Grace lived all over Texas, in Dallas, Granger, Marshall, Clarksville, Gilmer, and Daingerfield. On June 13, 1890, she was appointed as the first woman doctor to the staff at the North Texas State Hospital, in Terrell. She wrote articles for the publications *The Texas Sanitarian* and *The Texas Courier*. She was a renowned gynecologist of her time. Dr. Grace opposed homeopathy and spiritual cures, and she fought to gain equal status of all women.

Some sources say that at the time of her death, she was undergoing some severely depressing personal hardships, the nature of which has never been revealed. She was, however, known to be plagued with severe and debilitating headaches, which often hampered her medical practice because she refused to take anything for them. On that fateful night in February, she took a lethal dose of medicine.

Anyone who experiences cluster headaches knows the pain Grace experienced. A doctor once told me he had a patient who had cluster headaches. Doc thought the man merely wanted more narcotics, which he was obviously addicted to, so Doc told him that at the first sign of an oncoming headache to come to the office for some tests. The man showed up one Wednesday afternoon.

Doc hooked him up to every machine he had access to and told the man to stand the pain as long as he could so they could record, measure, and identify the source. The man did as told, or at least tried to. At first, he broke into a sweat, began breathing heavy, and just before he went in to convulsions, said softly, "Doc? Don't think I can take it much longer."

That man nearly destroyed over a hundred thousand dollars of equipment before Doc brought those convulsions under control. After that spell, whenever that man called and said he felt a headache coming on, Doc wrote him a prescription.

The problem with many modern painkillers, especially those that a physician can still phone in like the codeine derivative, hydrocodone, is that they lower the patient's pain threshold. What that means is, if a person normally has three debilitating headaches in a month, after a while the frequency could increase as tolerance develops to where it takes twice as much medicine to treat the same pain. On the other hand, if a person seldom takes narcotic pain medications, a large dose could be lethal. This type of patient is called *opiate naive.*

Another medication dosing problem is called *automatism.* Automatism is when a patient takes a dose of medicine, like a sleeping pill or pain medicine, wakes up later and forgets he took it, then takes another, and another and so forth until they either pass out or stop breathing.

It appears that since Dr. Grace Danforth was not one to take narcotics, or any drugs, for that matter, her demise was likely a combination of both automatism and opiate naiveté. She simply wasn't accustomed to the doses it took to relieve the headache she experienced that fateful night and died as a result.

Much wonderful advancement has been made in medicine since Grace Danforth's time. Sumatriptan succinate (Imitrex) and its analogs have brought amazing relief to severe headache sufferers. The doctor mentioned earlier tells me that the man who went into convulsions from a headache seldom takes narcotics any more; he takes shots of the new drugs. What a pity Dr. Grace Danforth didn't have access to such.

## GIVE ME A BREAK

In 1887, Dr. D. R. Fox, a southern doctor, treated a woman in labor. He delivered the child without incident, but during the night, the woman presented with a postpartum fever. Dr. Fox followed the medical protocol of the day and treated the condition by bleeding her of five units of blood (eighty ounces). That's a staggering amount when you consider that the average person has but ten units in his or her whole body. In addition, the good doctor dosed the poor girl with castor oil, gave her enough emetics to make her vomit every two hours, and then gave her an enema, likely via a clyster syringe—all within a twenty-four-hour period.

It took a month, but the woman fully recovered.

Bloodletting, laxatives, and enemas were pretty much the norm for all medical conditions in pioneer and frontier times. The enema itself usually contained herbs and assorted medicaments. The treatments themselves were gruesome enough, even worse when we look at the equipment used. Back then the two-foot-long hypodermic-looking clyster syringes were common instruments of misery (or relief, depending on how you look at it). (19—p. 43)

## A HOUSE OF PAIN

> Shinning tubercles of different size, dusky red or livid in color, on face, ears and extremities, together with a thickened and rugous state of the skin, a diminution or total loss of its sensibility, and a falling off of all hair except that of the scalp. . . .
>
> As the malady proceeds, the tubercles crack and ultimately ulcerate. Ulcerations also appear in the throat and nose, which sometimes destroy the palate and septum, the nose falls, and the breath is intolerably offensive; the fingers and toes gangrene, and separate joint after joint.

And so goes the Greek physician Aretacus of Cappadocia's description of leprosy. Leprosy was perhaps the most repulsing disease frontiersmen faced. But face it they did, not perhaps in epidemic proportions, but the problem often presented itself to early pioneers.

The disease was brought to the United States primarily by slave traffic and worldwide immigration that landed in New York and California and by French settlers who arrived in Louisiana. It was thought that some ships were loaded with lepers and sent to the Americas as a method of relieving their country of the disease. The Hawaiian Islands were a common dropping place for lepers.

Leprosy existed primarily in four of the continental states at the end of the nineteenth century: Florida, Texas, Louisiana, and California. Pioneers often mistook the festers of yaws, syphilis, and tuberculosis lesions on the skin as leprosy. Common Asians were capable of detecting leprosy at a glance. Early American physicians and pioneers, however, failed horribly in diagnosing the disease. For years people endured the stigma of having leprosy when in fact they didn't. One story has it that the citizens of a West Virginia town, having discovered what they thought was a leper, placed him in boxcar and nailed the door shut. This took place in the middle of winter. The man reportedly froze (and/or starved) to death before he was found many days later. There never was proof that he actually had the disease.

A Norwegian physician, Gerhard Armauer Hansen, in early 1870 proved that bacteria caused leprosy. Natives from India introduced the first drug used to treat leprosy to Americans, when they were seen chewing the leaves and twigs of the chaulmoogra tree to keep from getting the disease. It was later discovered that the oil from the plant's seeds contained the curative substance, chaulmoogra oil.

It wasn't until late in the nineteenth century, though, that any real progress, other than patient isolation, proved of benefit. Dr. Isadore Dyer, a professor of dermatology at Tulee University, brought Chaulmoogra oil to the attention of the scientific world in 1907 by presenting his successful treatment of cases at the Iverville Parish, Louisiana, colony of leprosy. However, the drugs benefits came with some serious drawbacks. The drug worked, but only if the patient could keep it down. Taken by mouth, most lepers became so nauseated that fewer than one in three hundred took it long enough to do any good. Many a poor leper made the statement that he'd rather have leprosy than take another dose of that horrible-tasting stuff.

Chaulmoogra oil was coated with everything imaginable to make it dissolve after it passed through the stomach (the equivalent of today's enteric-coated pills), but nothing worked back then. Enemas fortified with the oil were tried to no avail. Absolutely nothing made chaulmoogra tolerable. It wasn't until someone contacted Merck and Company in Germany to ask if there was any substance available which might cause chaulmoogra oil to be absorbed, that real progress in leprosy treatment was made. The use of hypodermics was coming into its own at the time the scientists at Merck reported that, theoretically, it was possible that if resorcin and camphor or ether were added to the oil and injected, it might work. To everyone's joy, the combination was readily absorbed. Shortly afterward, a number of cases negative of the leper bacilli were presented to the world.

Though slow, the drug did work. Literally thousands of lepers were released over time from their "disease-induced confinement." The only unsolved problem facing medicine was what to do about the disfiguration caused by the disease before it was cured.

In 1917, the United States Congress appropriated $250,000 for the construction of a hospital where all lepers could be cared for, rehabilitated, and reconstructed free of charge. The problem came in finding a place to build the hospital. Nobody wanted it near them.

Seventy miles from New Orleans, where since 1894 the inhabitants had sustained contact with tropical America, an Indian plantation existed as a place to isolate lepers. The government bought that plantation in Iberville Parish and erected the Carville Leprosarium, which was run by Dr. Oswald Denney. Most of the inhabitants of the hospital were Asian and Negroid Indian.

Leprosy itself was not normally painful. In some instances, it was even diagnosed by the patient's inability to "feel" anything in an infected extremity. Creoles were especially susceptible to a type of leprosy called *Leprous iritis*, the most agonizing of all leprosy infections. Laudanum and morphine could not be given in large enough doses to sufficiently eliminate the pain. Many patients afflicted with *Leprous iritis* begged daily to be killed.

The doctors at Carville did anything and everything to help the leper, to ease either the pain of their treatment or the social agony of being disfigured. Since leprosy often affects the bones and cartilage in the jaw, face, and extremities, some of the most elaborate artificial reproductions and restorations of the day were attempted. At Carville the patients were given the power to decide for themselves the treatments and reconstructive attempts undertaken on them, and they were allowed to stay as long as they wished.

Leprosy isn't a thing of the past. It still exists. Armadillos are known carriers of the leprosy bacteria. Texans joke about eating road-killed armadillo, when in fact few if any will even touch the little critters anymore. And rightly so.

## THE HAIR SHIRT

Malaria in the United States extended as far north as Wisconsin in pioneer days. In Washington at one point, swarms of mosquitoes interfered with sittings of Congress. Once the culprit that spread malaria was discovered to be a mosquito, draining surrounding land gradually helped slow the disease. In the nineteenth century, malaria was common in Connecticut where some Italian immigrants with the infection in their blood had swarmed from abroad to settle the land. Railroad embankments, irrigation, and the early development of roads in the South during this period created perfect artificial breeding grounds for the mosquito.

In a demonstration in Crossett, Arkansas, a project was undertaken to prove that a town could be free of malaria by eliminating mosquitoes and their habitat. The project was a success, but many theories were upset by this experiment. The main focus after that was to determine which mosquito carried the disease. The *anopheles* was known as a vector, but over thirty species had already been discovered. It was well known that in the Philippines only one or two of the anopheles species were an important factor in malaria transmission. Furthermore, a species of danger in one foreign country might not be a danger in another. It wasn't until it 1883 that it was discovered that something carried by individual anopheles mosquitoes caused the disease, not the mosquito itself.

Major education campaigns were undertaken to help eradicate the anopheles mosquito's habitat. There was a minnow called the Texas gambusia, which was capable of living equally well in salt, fresh, running, or stagnant water. The little minnow was a ferocious eater of mosquito "wigglers" and was even transported to other states and abroad in hopes it might propagate and help control malaria.

During the late nineteenth and early twentieth centuries, an arsenic compound, aceto-arsenite of copper, also called Paris green, was used to help eliminate mosquitoes. The compound was mixed with ninety-nine parts of powdery sand and spread over streams and ponds. It was so effective that if the dust was poured from one container to another in the same room with a dish full of wigglers, it killed the larvae within minutes. A benefit that Paris green had over pouring oil on water to kill mosquito larvae was that water treated with it could be drunk or used in any manner without harm to the consumer.

Pouring petroleum oil on water to control mosquito larvae had its advantages and disadvantages. Granted, the water couldn't be consumed, but some species of the mosquito larvae didn't feed on the surface where Paris green floated (the wiggler had to consume the chemical to work). One species of anopheles mosquito, the *Culex* larva, fed with its head hanging below the surface and ate only particles suspended in the water. A thin film of oil prevented any and all mosquitoes from obtaining air. Oil itself was expensive even back then and was ineffective on moving water. Still, pouring a thin film of oil, rancid bacon grease, petroleum, or anything like it on the surface of water became the preferred method for a frontiersman to help eliminate the malaria-carrying mosquito's breeding places.

A friend from Louisiana tells me that in the southern part of that state, somewhere near New Iberia, I think he said, Cajuns gather to eat, drink, party, and drink some more, and have a "toughest man" contest. The contestants supposedly gather in late evening in a swamp where mosquitoes are so thick a person can't breathe. At the drop of a flag, the contestants remove their shirts and squat at the water's edge. The last man to jump in the water wins. I'm told that within minutes every contestant's back looks like he was wearing a hair shirt. Just the thought of that makes my back itch. My friend said, too, that they were opening the contest to everyone next year, men and women. I told him thanks anyway for the invite, but I had absolutely no intentions of ever getting that drunk.

## A TRUE, INSIDE GLANCE AT INDIGESTION

When William Beaumont left home in 1806 on a horse and set out to conquer the world, he never knew he would become famous. He taught school for a while before deciding to become a doctor. For two years he served as an apprentice with a practicing physician, enlisted in the army, and became an assistant surgeon in the War of 1812. One day, while in a store replenishing his food supplies, a gun was accidentally discharged into a French Canadian's stomach. The shot man's name was Alexis St. Martin.

Although it seemed impossible to save the gut-shot man, Beaumont tended him. St. Martin's wound healed but never fully sealed itself. It had a flap of flesh that hung over the hole, which was kind of like a colostomy opening directly into the stomach. Raise the flap, and you got a glimpse of his shiny and juicy insides. Dr. Beaumont took advantage of the chance to watch digestion in action as he nursed St. Martin. He noted the rate at which the stomach emptied, how long it took certain foods to digest; he collected samples of various states of digested contents and examined them. Firsthand, he studied the effect alcohol had on the stomach and the digestive juices.

Alexis St. Martin died at the age of eighty-four, and Dr. William Beaumont died at the age of sixty-eight, but not before publishing in 1833 his famous work, *Experiments and Observations on the Gastric Juice and the Physiology of Digestion*. This publication established the basis for present-day knowledge of the working stomach and its digestive processes. (40–p. 340)

## BLOODLETTING

Recently, after having read to a writer's group a chapter from a novel I'm writing, one man critiquing my 1870-based story cautioned me on using "present-day" teachings on artificial respiration. While doing my research for this book, I ran across an interesting article about bloodletting, which appeared in 1812. Following the article was this piece:

> Let a person of good strong lungs apply his mouth to the sufferer's holding at the same time his nostrils and blow his breath as hard as he can into the sufferer's lungs; he must then leave him to expire while he gets his own breath, and then repeat the effort as soon and as often as he can, perhaps a hundred times, if self-respiration does not take place sooner.

I went home the night after that critique and changed my story in that novel; but I'm going back and redo it to its original draft. All I can say to that critic is, "Th! Th! Th! Th! Th!"

Anyway, before chloroform came into being, a healthy imbibing of whiskey was the only thing available to get a "slow" gunfighter through the removal of a poorly aimed projectile. But gritting one's teeth, or biting the old bullet, didn't start with John Wayne; it began long before he was born.

All one has to do is look at a nineteenth-century surgical kit to imagine the gruesome pain that injured pioneers suffered. I'm afraid that by the standards of people who lived in the nineteenth century, I'd be classified as a *thumb-thuckin' wussy*. Just thinking about having my arm amputated, or doing it myself, as was reported recently, or having a doctor probe me for a bullet with a pair of needle-nosed pliers, or bleeding me like a hog, sends chill bumps up my spine. If I can't go to a hospital and have total anesthesia, I'd die of anticipation.

There were only two hospitals in all of America in 1800. The first was Pennsylvania Hospital in Philadelphia, which began in 1751; the other was New York Hospital, founded in 1771.

Bloodletting was a popular medical technique back then. No doubt a person with high blood pressure felt better after a treatment. One positive aspect of bloodletting was when treating a person who ate too much meat. Diets heavy in red meats have been proven to cause a condition called "iron overload," which is thought to relate to coronary occlusion (stopped-up veins and arteries in the heart). Bleeding unknowingly helped alleviate iron overload. Using it for anything else doesn't make sense.

There were two types of bloodletting used in pioneer days. The first was opening of a vein (venisection) or an artery (arteriotomy) and letting the blood run freely into a measured container; the second was by a suction process (sanguisuction) using a bulb or other convenient leeching or cupping device. Many of the instruments used spring-loaded blades to open the blood vessel.

Lewis and Clark used bloodletting routinely on their expedition in the early 1800s.

Even as early as 1835, a French physician named Pierre Louis statistically analyzed bloodletting and decided it was all but a useless medical process. But old habits were hard to break. The practice was slow to die in the old west.

A sanguisuction bloodletting procedure that hasn't gone away is leeches. For thousands of years the little "blood suckers from the creeks" had been used to medically remove blood from the human body. Leeches have a sucker at each end of their bodies. The mouth end has row upon row of teeth that the leech uses to attach itself to its host. Aside from being used to simply remove blood (a leech consumes up to five times its own weight in blood), leeches were used to remove black eyes or facial hematomas (blood under the skin) by sucking out the stagnant blood.

They had other benefits, too. Along with an anesthetic that makes their biting attachment and sucking processes painless, the saliva of a leech contains *hirudin*, an organic compound that prevents blood from clotting. We recently had a patient at the hospital where I work. The child had had her hand mashed nearly off. The prognosis after surgery didn't look good, so the attending physician had leeches flown in that were attached to her fingers. Almost immediately her tiny blue fingernails turned pink as the components of the leech saliva began to increase circulation and dissolve blood clots. Thanks to those leeches, the child didn't lose those fingers. The local anesthetic the yucky-looking little critters pumped into her hand made the process totally painless, too. (19–p. 9; 47–accessed September 6, 2002)

## THE WORMS CRAWL IN . . .

The slave trade in America's formative years was big business. Abroad, innocent natives were ambushed, bound and gagged, and placed on ships and brought to the United States where they were sold into bondage. With these slaves came new diseases and conditions Americans had never before encountered, one being a ghastly disease called *dracunculiasis* (dra-kunk-you-lie-uh-sis), a parasitic infection caused by *Dracunculus medinensis*, better known as the guinea worm. Slaves captured and brought particularly from Africa acquired the parasite by drinking water contaminated with "water fleas." The larva of the guinea worm was swallowed by the small copepods and matured inside the insect. Anyone consuming water that contained the near-microscopic water fleas became infected.

The worm was released from the flea by digestive juices inside the person's stomach. During the year following exposure (about the time it took to transport a slave to the United States), the worm migrated to the surface of the body where it released chemicals into the skin and caused blisters, out of which it stuck its head. Guinea worms literally popped out anywhere—the mouth, torso, legs, and buttocks. An infected person who entered water of any kind gave the worm the opportunity to cough up a milky fluid containing millions of immature worms, thus contaminating yet another water source.

Once the worm's head emerged from the wound, it could be pulled out over a period weeks depending on its length by wrapping the head around a stick and making a wind or two every few

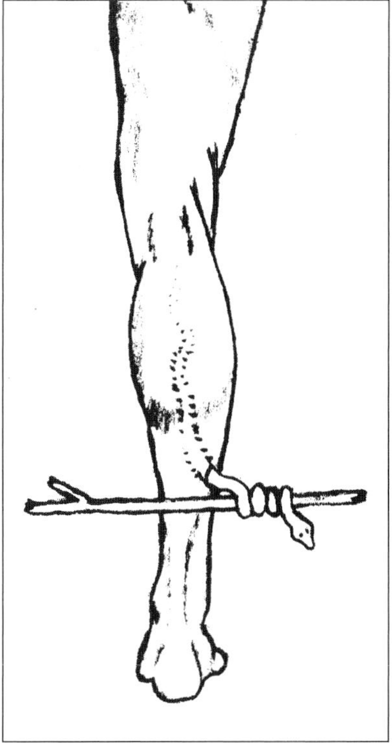

*Guinea worm being rolled onto a stick*

days. Some guinea worms grew three feet in length and hid beneath the skin like a tapered blood vein. Pulling it out more than a few centimeters a day caused the worm to break in two and release toxins, which killed its host within days.

Sounds like a nightmare straight off of Frontier Elm Street, but unfortunately, dracunculiasis still exists today in thirteen countries in Africa, primarily between the Sahara and the equator where in remote areas people still drink contaminated water. More than a thousand cases a year are reported.

Ironically, in the past century we put a man on the moon, but we can't eradicate the guinea worm. There are still no known medications to prevent or stop the instant death from the toxins released if the worm breaks inside the body. Doing surgery to remove the worm intact, drinking clean water, preventing persons known to be infected from entering ponds and streams used for drinking, filtering out the water fleas, and treating the water with a product known as Abate, which kills the insects that carry the worm's larvae, are the only known treatments.

You don't reckon this is where the old saying "Do at least one good turn a day" comes from, do you?

Maggots, too, turn man's stomach. But they did man good, believe it or not. Also known as living antiseptic, the larvae of the green fly have been used for centuries to remove necrotic (dead) material. The maggot serves as nature's street sweeper. Whether it be a wound from a cannon ball, saber cut, or the gore of an ox or milk cow, flies were allowed (sometimes willingly, sometimes not) to blow the wound, and the little grubs left to do their work for several days or until the wound became moist with fresh blood. Maggots improve healing in gross wounds by secreting enzymes that liquefy dead tissue, enzymes (collogenase, for one) that are known to have antibacterial activity. The fluids thus formed while they "wove in and out" helped wash the wound. Urea, allantoin, calcium, and ammonium compounds in the maggot's secretions promoted healing.

The heightened physical activity of the worm (the playing of pinochle on your snout, so to speak) stimulates circulation to the wound and activates the body's own defense mechanisms. Also contained in the larvae's excrement are growth-stimulating hormonal factors.

Green fly maggots devour only dead tissue. They do not reproduce in the wound, nor do mature flies mature in the wound. Once the dead tissue was removed, the wound was flushed (the worms were made to crawl out, as the old poem goes) with a balanced saline solution. I had a buddy who served in Vietnam who stepped on a land mine and lay a long time before being flown out. Maggots got in the wound in his arm and were left there until he could be evacuated to a hospital and removed. To this day, occasionally, a phantom wiggling and tickling in his elbow wakes him up at night.

Frontiersmen got worms inside them in other ways, too. The hookworm is a nematode called *Ancylostoma duodenale* that lives inside a human by attaching itself to the intestines with little hooks. The larva of the hookworm, which lives in moist dirt, enters the skin through a scratch or sore on the sole of a person's foot and hitches a ride in the bloodstream to the lungs. There it causes festering and coughing and a bloody discharge created solely as a vehicle to get hacked to the back of the throat where it gets swallowed. The larva slide down the gut and by means of little "hooks" attaches to the upper portion of the small intestine, where it feasts on its host's blood. A mature female can produce as many as thirty thousand eggs that are passed in the feces, and the cycle starts all over. Hookworms in number drink so much blood from their host that they cause anemia.

Large armies of men amassed during the Civil War spread the disease in epidemic proportions, thanks to camp sanitation and going barefoot, especially around water holes where baths were taken and where defecating in the bushes nearby was common. The larvae lay in wait for an unsuspecting host with a sore on their foot. The army's inability to provide shoes made barefoot soldiers easy prey.

Hookworms sapped so much blood from their hosts that they created a state of apathetic laziness in the troops. Some were so anemic they appeared mentally retarded. A number of folk treatments were tried—iron supplementation via tonics and various vermifuge concoctions containing pomegranate, turpentine, licorice, and castor and croton oil. The best medicine of all was prevention by proper sanitation and the wearing of shoes.

It wasn't until tetrachloroethylene was synthesized by Michael Faraday in 1821 that any real cure for hookworm was found. Tetrachloroethylene made the worms "unhook" from the gut, die, and pass from the body. By 1920, the drug's most significant use was commercially as a solvent for cleaning and degreasing. One might say that tetrachloroethylene, in tiny doses, "dry-cleaned" the hookworms from the gut. The chemical is still employed as a solvent by 80 to 90 percent of today's dry cleaners. Because of its toxicity and difficult administration, here in the States, anyway, tetrachloroethylene has been replaced by newer, safer medications like mebendazole (Vermox).

Roundworms, *Ascaris lumbricoides*, are very similar to earthworms that have tapered ends. They reach a length of six to ten inches. When passed from the bowel, they appear yellowish in color and somewhat transparent. Normally they don't infect children less that two or three years of age. Roundworms reside in the small intestine of their host and can reach quantities of well over a hundred at a time. In larger numbers like that, they form themselves into a ball in the gut. Yet, even in mass they caused little pain or discomfort other than a "tickling" sensation now and then or a sense of bloat. Diagnosis occurred when an exploring worm or two ventured too low in the gut and got passed with a bowel movement brought on by a large-dose purgative or cathartic. The most common treatment was six to eight grains of pinkroot in castor oil or senna that was given in hourly doses until the feces presented clear of worms. A common recipe was to place two tablespoonfuls each of powdered pinkroot and senna leaves into a pint of boiling water and letting the concoction steep several hours before being strained through thin muslin. A teaspoonful of rectified turpentine and/or two ounces of castor oil were added. The mixture was bottled and dosed at a tablespoonful every hour. Reportedly, the taste was almost not worth the gain.

The pinworm was a small round worm, *Enterobius vermicularis*, and was the most common source of human worm infection in frontier days. Children were more commonly infested than adults. The little worm congregated, mated, and lived in the large intestine. Mature females migrated to the anus where they deposited literally tens of thousands of eggs. Within a matter of hours they began to spread by contact. Contamination took place by handling previously touched household objects or foods.

The life cycle of the pinworm was two to six weeks. Live eggs could live up to three weeks in warm environments. Once swallowed, they hatched in the upper gut and then migrated to the lower bowel, where the cycle began all over again. Seeing a child scratch his rear, astronomically, or scoot on the floor like a dog, was a sure-fire indication that they had pinworms. Cleanliness and strict personal hygiene, washing hands and body (particularly the rear end), and boiling bed linens and clothing were the best measures to control the spread of pinworms. Oral treatment was combined with purgation before, during, and after by administering a vermifuge. Cathartics like croton oil, cascara, and senna helped "push" the worms out.

A ten- to fourteen-day round with remedies containing rectified turpentine, pomegranate, pumpkin seeds, garlic, and gentian violet were the accepted treatments of frontier physicians and pioneer doctor-moms. Many of the little worms, in their attempt to "get the hell outta here," were expelled alive. After having taken gentian violet to move 'em out, one can't help but imagine what that squirming, purple mess looked like in an old two-holer. "Hey, guys, come look at this!"

Because of its supposed carcinogenic possibilities, gentian violet is no longer used as a vermifuge for pinworms. Safer, one-dose therapies like mebendazole have taken their place.

Untreated abdominal worm infestations, as many cases were in frontier times, by sheer volume could give a person a "pot gut." The nutritional drain the parasites put on the body made the person look drawn and dark beneath the eyes. This is where the old expression "He sure looks wormy" comes from.

Tapeworms that plagued the frontiersman came in several varieties. There was the *Taenia saginata,* or beef tapeworm; the *Taenia solium,* or pork tapeworm; *Bothriocephalus latus,* from fish; *Hymenolepsis nana,* or dwarf tapeworm; which was transmitted through fecal (poop) contamination and was common in children in the southern United States. Then there was the *Echinoccus granulosis,* which spent its adult phase in the intestine of dogs.

Humans got the tapeworm by eating undercooked, infested

meat. History shows that people contracted this parasite thousands of years ago from game that was eaten raw. Antelopes were known carriers, as well as the pigs, cows, dogs, and fish mentioned.

Many medicines were used to treat tapeworms: calomel, worm seed oil, Carolina and Indian pinkroot, aloe vera juice mixed with honey. A tea made from pinkroot by boiling a handful in a quart of water, adding sugar, milk, and castor oil did the job quite well—too well on occasion. Sometimes the pinkroot was detrimental to the patient; its causing sore eyes was an indication of poisoning the body far beyond its ability to eject the worm. Sore eyes meant it was time to start giving the patient charcoal mixed in milk to help "rescue" the person's health.

In pharmacy school, during pharmacognosy class one day, Dr. C. C. Albers told us about a man who purposely infected himself with a tapeworm and let it mature. His reason for doing so was purely medicinal. For one, he was overweight. The worm would share his food consumption and help keep his weight down. Second, but more important, he was going abroad to study drugs used in underdeveloped countries. His theory was that he could eat and drink anything he wished while traveling in a country where water and food were known to cause "Montezuma's revenge." The worm worked. The man spent his entire trip eating and drinking anything he wanted with absolutely no ill effects. He said he could even drink stagnant water if necessary. When he returned to the States, he treated himself to remove the worm and lived happily ever after.

Many natural, fast-running streams from the purest mountain waters were contaminated with worms back in frontier times—not only with *Giardia* (an infestation of a flagellate protozoan, *Giardia lamblia*, that is often characterized by diarrhea) but with some nasty little creatures most people have never heard about—that brought on conditions like "clam diggers itch" or "lakeside disease" or "swimmer's itch." These are all names for an infestation of the skin with a little booger known as *Schistosome* (be careful how you pronounce that), a larva that was a parasitic flatworm that plagued people living in many midwestern lake areas, the coastal water areas of the Northeast, the Gulf of Mexico, and the Pacific Northwest. People got it by wading or swimming in infested lakes and streams. The adult form of this worm came from infected birds and animals. The worm's eggs passed into the stools of these animals, got into the water, and hitched a ride inside snails, where they matured into vicious little swimmers that cruised the waters looking for other birds or animals or people to attack. The parasite, fortunately, did not penetrate healthy human skin, so it set up shop on tender skin and created an intensely itchy and bumpy red rash that whelped up and spread across legs and body and other tender body parts. The rash usually peaked after a few days and then slowly subsided after a couple of weeks. Treatment was symptomatic: applying turpentine, moonshine, vinegar, or sulfur mixed in axel grease. Since the parasite needed to remain on the skin a while before propagating, drying off immediately when exiting the water was the best way to prevent its taking hold. Unfortunately, most old-timers dripped dry to enjoy the wonderful coolness of their once-a-year bath, and they ended up with a maddening rash that developed a few days later.

This swimmer's itch was usually not terminal, just maddening. But there is a more deadly little critter that infected warm water springs—one that did and still will kill. It's called *Naegleria foweri,* an amoeba that infests natural hot springs where it breeds year-round. It enters the body through mucous membranes in the nose and attacks the brain. Fever and headaches and aching begin within days before coma and death set in.

An infection of the *N. foweri* amoeba undoubtedly accounted for many frontiersman's "mysterious" deaths after bathing in hot, natural springs. Even today, by the time an infection of *N. foweri* is diagnosed, it's too late. The only real remedy is to avoid these waters. Unfortunately, pioneers didn't know about it, and many died as a result. Some old-timers thought that bathing too much could kill ya. They were right.

In all my research for this piece, I found worms that crawled in, some that crawled out, some that ate flesh of the eyes, ears, and snout, but as yet, I find no evidence of a worm that eats the goody from between your toes. (4; 18–p. 430–37; 48–accessed August 27, 2002; 49–accessed September 4, 2002)

## WHO'S THERE?

The advent of anesthetics opened the way for modern surgery as early as 1840, but real anesthesia's use in an operation didn't occur until 1846 at the Massachusetts General Hospital. Painless or not, most patients died anyway. It seemed that the longer a surgery took, the more likely a patient was to die from a "mysterious poison" in the air. Here is a story about that mysterious poison in the air.

Outside, the night sounds were haunting, an Oregon winter wind whined in the background, its normal ebb and flow rising and falling in an eerie wail; snow swirled softly, falling in ghostly silence on the windowpane. Bethenia snuggled her nose into her feather pillow and sighed. It had been a long day, too long. She could finally rest. The down comforter felt good against her cheek as she sighed into it. She'd no sooner drifted off before a lantern swayed outside her window and voice called out, "Dr. Owens? Dr. Owens?"

"Who is it?"

A man's face, pale with panic, came into view. Snow covered his whiskers; ice plastered his mustache. "It's my wife. Can you please come?" he yelled through the window, his breath blowing puffs of quickly dissipating fog on the cold pane.

She threw on some clothes and threaded her arms into her coat. Black bag in hand, she hurried out into the storm. As they walked she continually questioned the man. It didn't sound good.

The year was 1896; Bethenia had just gotten back from Chicago where she'd studied a new surgical procedure. She'd heard previously of appendectomies being done, but she'd never seen one performed. She witnessed that and her first operation on a heart while in Chicago. In her years of doing surgery, she had lost many patients to appendicitis. Finally there was something that could be done.

Bethenia's fear became reality when she examined the suffering woman. Afraid the appendix would rupture if they moved her to town in a wagon, she turned to the man and said, "I must remove it at once."

He glanced across the room, wiped his hand across his mouth, and replied, "I don't want you to operate."

"It's either that, or she'll die." She then turned and said with authority, "Build a big fire in the stove, fill that boiler with water, and boil it while I prepare her. Help me get her on the table."

With her forceful takeover and firm commands, the man did as told.

The light was much too dim, but it would have to do. She boiled her surgical instruments in a dishpan, placed everything in order on clean linens within easy reach, carefully exposed the woman's abdomen, and sprayed it with carbolic acid. "You'll have to do the anesthesia, while I operate. Pour a little of that ether there onto this cloth and hold it over her nose. Stop when I say, and pour more on when I say." The man reluctantly did as told.

Bethenia had studied Joseph Lister's work on the importance of sterile procedure. She scrubbed her hands well and applied carbolic acid and touched the tissues with only freshly boiled instruments. Skillfully, just as she'd seen done in Chicago, the incision was made. She carefully located and gently snipped the perforated appendix from the gut, removed it, stitched where it had been attached, and sewed the abdomen back up.

A week or so later she came to check on the woman's progress. Hat in hand, the husband approached. "I didn't want no woman cuttin' up my wife. But if you hadn't manhandled me, she'd be dead. Thanks, doctor."

That was the way Dr. Bethenia Owens-Adair (1840–1926), the

first woman surgeon in Oregon, came to do her first appendectomy. This story is also the first documentation I could find of any woman surgeon performing an appendectomy.

Bethenia Owens-Adair began her medical training in 1874 at the Eclectic Medical College in Philadelphia. She completed her surgical training at the University of Michigan Medical School in 1880. She was also known for her position on mandatory sterilization for the criminally insane. Because of her continued support and efforts, in 1925, a sterilization statue was adopted into law by the Oregon legislature.

Bethenia was another of the dedicated, persistent women who made a serious difference in the progress of frontier medicine. During her practice, she admired and studied under a skillful male physician named Dr. Roderick McLean. On one occasion she asked him, "Don't you think there might be something to this Lister theory of keeping wounds clean from germs with carbolic acid spray while operating?"

Dr. McLean's reply was, "Balderdash! Keep the wound clean by operating fast." (35; 43–pp. 122, 157; 49)

## WATER CURES

Water as a medicine? Git serious!

Recently, my wife and I stopped at a convenience store. I was thirsty; so was my truck. As I filled the gas tank, my wife walked up and handed me a moisture-fogged bottle of the best double-filtered, reverse-osmosis cold water I ever tasted. She went back inside to pick up a few more items—we were out of milk. We knew the price was too high here, but we were ready to get home. Fishing wears a person out. As I sipped my water and pumped my gas, a cute "Got milk?" ad caught my attention. I looked at the price of the milk, over at the price of the gas, and then down at the price tag on the bottle in my hand. Did you ever think you'd see the day when water cost more per gallon than either milk or gasoline?

Dehydration is an interesting process. Once when I was consulting at a nursing home, a salesman came by my drugstore with a trunk full of Gatorade, the packages of which had gotten wet during shipping and were unsellable. He donated the whole lot to the nursing home next door. Given access to the free liquid, some residents who normally sat around in various states of gloom, after filling themselves on the liquids, got up and walked around, visiting and laughing.

Chronic dehydration creates a state of lethargy. Thirst, the body's alarm system, is a poor indicator of bodily fluid levels. By the time the body reacts, it's already several pints too low. If the back of the hand of a dehydrated person is pinched, the tissue remains pinched for a few moments, signifying fluid depletion.

Few people consume the recommended eight glasses of "plain" water a day and exist in a chronic state of near-dehydration. Think about it; the first thing done when a person is admitted to the hospital is to be put on an IV to restore fluid volume. They are now trying to relate heart problems with chronic dehydration. It appears that the earlobes of most heart attack victims are creased in a horizontal line, like they've been folded down the middle. It does make sense that if the skin on the back of one's hand remains fixed when pinched to reflect acute dehydration that deep creases in a heart attack victim's earlobes reflects years of insufficient fluid consumption or chronic dehydration.

A branch of medicine called *homeopathy* bases its practices on the *potentization* and *dynamization* of water. Patients are hydrated, and then treated with homeopathic medicines. These "water cure" medicines are prepared by diluting medications serially in pure water in a process called *succession*, which is little more than vigorous shaking. Several fundamentally sound, medically recognized principles are based on this homeopathic theory that small doses stimulate and large doses inhibit physiological action. For example, similar medicines in minute doses are the basis for the desensitization processes used by today's most respected allergists. The concept of

Don't miss sales by running out of CRAZY WATER CRYSTALS. You'll find it pays to always have it when your customers demand this old favorite of millions for over 70 years.

Keep your stocks of

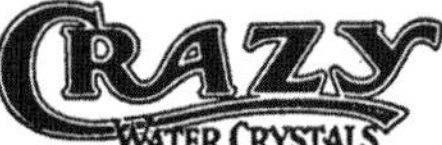


and other Crazy Water Company products up at all times

**Regular CRAZY CRYSTALS**

a household word in thousands of homes for quick, pleasant relief from many ailments due to excess gastric acidity and constipation.

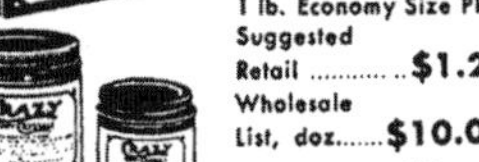

1 lb. Economy Size Pkg.
Suggested Retail ........ **$1.25**
Wholesale List, doz....... **$10.00**

½ lb. Regular Size Pkg.
Suggested Retail.................. **85¢**
Wholesale List, doz....... **$6.80**

**Powdered CRAZY CRYSTALS**

6 oz. Economy Size Jar
Suggested Retail................ **75¢**
Wholesale List, doz.......... **$6.00**

3 oz. Regular Size Jar
Suggested Retail.............. **40¢**
Wholesale List, doz......... **$3.20**

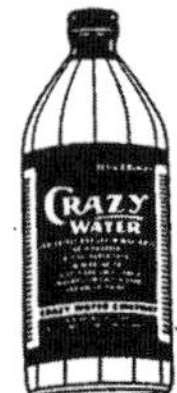


**CRAZY WATER**

Direct from the famous wells of Mineral Wells, Texas, in refined concentrated form.

1 Quart Size
Suggested Retail ............ **$1.50**
Wholesale List, doz....... **$12.00**

**OXIDINE for malaria**

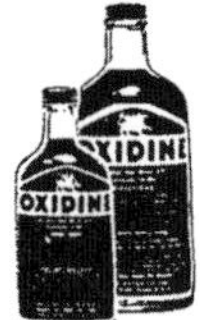


An old time specific treatment for chills and fever, aches and pains due to Malaria. Directions printed in English and Spanish.

4 oz. Size
Suggested Retail ............... **75¢**
Wholesale List, doz.......... **$6.00**

10 oz. Size
Suggested Retail ............ **$1.25**
Wholesale List, doz....... **$10.00**

**NEXT *Brushless* Shave Cream**

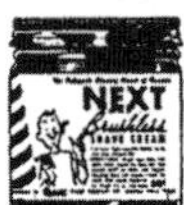


Men appreciate the extra smoothness of NEXT triple whip texture for the smartest shave they've ever had.

Regular Size 5½ oz.
Suggested Retail......... **50¢** Wholesale List, doz. **$4.00**

***Order these products from your wholesaler, NOW!***

CRAZY WATER CO., INC., Mineral Wells, Texas

vaccination is also based on activating the body to respond on its own to diseases by injecting tiny amounts of the causative agent.

There used to be an old poison ivy preventive treatment on the market that was little more than a weak solution of poison ivy juice. It was dosed by placing two drops in a glass of purified water and drinking it daily for a week, three drops daily for a week, and so on, until twenty drops a day were reached. By the end of the treatment period, the patient would be immune to poison ivy. The "immunization" it afforded worked; the problem came at the end of the therapy when the irritating ingredient, *urishiol*, passed into the feces and a maddening anal rash that most people couldn't handle presented itself.

From a purely scientific perspective, homeopathy appears to be illogical at best and nonsensical at worst. Criticism is especially true when drugs are diluted beyond twenty-four times (decimally), since these dilutions far surpass the properties of the original substance's medical value. Ironically, double-blind studies (studies in which neither doctor nor patient knows what medicine is being given, the gold standard for evaluating a medicine's worth) have provided rational foundations for the healing phenomenon involved in using minute dilutions as practiced by homeopathic physicians.

In 1870, a doctor named Sylvester Andral Kilmer studied homeopathy, which at the time (and still is) thought to be a bunch of hogwash. He prepared many different medicines, some of which his colleagues said were pure bunk. His best-known remedy, which wasn't truly homeopathic, was a theriac (cure-all) that is still available on drugstore shelves nationwide. Kilmer's remedy contained buchu leaves, oil of juniper, oil of birch, colombo root, balsam copaiba, balsam tolu, skullcap leaves, Venice turpentine, valerian root, rhubarb root, mandrake root, peppermint herb, aloes, cinnamon and sugar, and swamp sassafras, all in a 10 percent (20 proof) alcohol base.

Dr. Kilmer named his concoction Swamp Root Kidney Liver and Bladder Cure. Willis Kilmer, heir to the swamp root legacy, was once asked what swamp root really was good for. He laughed and said, "About a million dollars a year." Dr. Kilmer's old swamp root remedy is still made and sold—and used with success by Texans—to this very day.

In 1892, the good doctor Kilmer sold his interests in his Swamp Root Remedies and constructed a cancertorium, where he advocated homeopathic treatment of cancer. Keep in mind here that Dr. Kilmer was fully trained in the practices of the modern medical and surgical techniques of the day. His practice of homeopathy was under constant scrutiny by his colleagues, and when he tried to share his successful findings, he was scoffed. The cancer patients Kilmer treated held him in the highest regard and flocked to his center from all over the world. Whether or not his cancer cure worked is still open to conjecture, but when his distant relative, John E. Golley, was asked in 1997 if Kilmer's homeopathic cancer treatments really worked, he said that his grandmother and sister would have both answered with a resolute yes.

Sylvester Andral Kilmer, M.D., ridiculed by his peers and scoffed by science, took his secret cancer cure to the grave with him on January 14, 1924. One can't help but wonder, what if?

Some western waters were thought in the nineteenth century to have direct curing properties. In December 1877, a man by the name of James Alvis Lynch, in search of a drier, healthier climate than his Red River Valley farm near Denison, Texas, moved to and settled about a good day's horseback ride southwest to near what is known today as Graham, Texas. Lynch was unable to find drinking water, so he and his family hauled it from the Brazos River. One day he decided to dig a well, but the water he found tasted funny. At first he thought it might be poison. For days he and his wife sipped and tested the "salty" water to see if made them sick. It didn't. In fact, drinking it cured his wife's rheumatism, the cause for their leaving the muggy malarial bottomlands back in Denison in the first place. This "medical water's" curative effects he shared with his neighbors. News of how drinking it helped cure all kinds of ills spread quickly. Soon, people flocked to his mineral well. Scores of ailing patients reportedly arrived on stretchers and left on foot.

It was once said that if a sane and healthy man walked upright to the well and drank, he left slumped over and walking sideways. In contrast, it was said that if a crazy person who normally walked sideways and slump shouldered approached and drank, they walked straight away, erect of back, and sane of mind.

The healthy people drank it because after they got over the water's "hangover" effects, they felt wonderful—and they did, but it could have simply been that they were dehydrated to start with or just needed a good bowel movement. Many folk remedies were based on the old theory that if it didn't hurt, or make you "feel it," or move you, it wasn't healing you.

The town of Mineral Wells sprang up as time passed. Bathhouses were erected, and the area became a quiet respite for the sick and even the insane. Life was very casual. Residents and visitors alike bathed in the waters, played dominoes, took long walks, rode "nightingales," and just relaxed letting the curative powers of the water do its job. (Nightingales, by the way, were Mineral Wells's famous mules that got the name from their high-pitched voices.) The town at night took on a Bourbon Street atmosphere. Hotels were built that staged music concerts and vaudeville acts; "beauty" doctors, fortune-tellers, and fakirs selling lotions and snake oils caroused the crowds.

It wasn't long before crystals were extracted from the water so patients could take the "magic" home with them and turn their own drinking water in to a healing potion. The consumer was instructed to dissolve the crystals in eight ounces of water and drink up to eight glasses a day. Take note that eight glasses a day is today's recommended treatment to prevent chronic dehydration; here the water might have had as much medical significance as the salts in it. This treatment was touted as a remedy for urticaria, cirrhosis of the liver, diabetes, gallstones, rheumatism, arthritis, high blood pressure—you name it, the crazy crystals were said to cure it. The main ingredient in the water turned out to be little more than Glauber's salt, a form of Epsom salt, the same laxative Lewis and Clark took on their famous expedition. However, there was another interesting ingredient in this water that did help cure the crazy people. It was lithium, a natural element, which is still used today to treat manic depression.

Mineral springs and their "curative ablutions" were very popular in the nineteenth century. The town of Mineral Wells, Texas, because of its crazy crystal fame, is the first that comes to mind, but by and far, it wasn't the first and only famous healing spot.

On Texas State Highway 49, less than a two-hour steam-engine train ride northwest of Shreveport, sits a small town that in 1839 was called Chalybeate Springs. A man named Reese Hughes settled and built a cabin beside the three springs where "funny-tasting" water gushed from the ground. In 1854, Hughes also constructed one of the nation's first blast furnaces to harvest native ore abundant in the area. His pig-iron foundry was seized by the Confederacy in 1862. The Union confiscated the foundry in 1866 and destroyed it. Hughes never received a cent for his loss.

The popularity of his chalybeate springs was his salvation. He and his wife, Elizabeth, built a four-story English-style castle, which became a renowned focal health spot for the not so fit and ailing. In Reese's honor, the community was later renamed Hughes Springs. In 1876, the East Line and Red River Railroad built its way beside the town. Sawmills, cotton gins, churches, a school, farming, and easy access to shipping helped the town grow. By 1878, Hughes Springs had become a flourishing health resort to which people flocked from all over the world to be revitalized by the spring's "magic" powers. The minerals in the springs, mostly iron carbonates, did indeed make those who drank it feel, "by Gawd, much better."

One visiting the springs back then would have thought the town's population would exceed thousands. The count of a mere three hundred permanent residents remained relatively stable during the 1800s, but by the early twentieth century, the government's attacking cure-all remedies, farming becoming more diversified, and the railroad terminus extending farther west saw to the town's demise. For a town that depended heavily on being a healthful place to visit, it rapidly became little more than a wide spot in the road to somewhere else. By the way, another "little" foundry was built near there to harvest the abundant iron ore. The monstrous Lone Star Steel Company is still in operation.

The old hotel and the English-style mansion are long gone, but you can still get in tune with the past, snag a precious moment in time, and sample the funny-tasting water of those once famous chalybeate springs. Spring Park, which was established in 1880, still stands. Just off the main highway (ask anyone there where it is), a full city block has been set aside for the mineral-rich springs that still trickle from the old concrete-covered cisterns. And today, by Gawd, you can drink from it free—compliments of Mother Nature and the friendly residents of Hughes Springs, Texas.

In 1884, a blacksmith named Matt Rains burned his hand and reportedly applied water from a "curative" well in Tioga, Texas, a community some forty miles due north of Fort Worth. Railroad workers who stopped to drink at the well discovered Tioga and its miraculously healing waters. Daily life in Tioga centered on bathing activities. Records show that ten trainloads of people a day flocked to Tioga to get healed. In the early part of the twentieth century, an unsuccessful effort was made to change Tioga's name to Autry Springs, Texas, in honor of a man who was born there. Tioga was the birthplace and hometown of none other than the famous singing cowboy, Gene Autry. Autry's family came to the area in covered wagons. His grandfathers helped settle the town of Tioga.

The now-abandoned area in the northwestern corner of Robertson County between Bremond and the Brazos River (thirty-five miles south east of Waco), back in the mid-nineteenth century, was another thriving Texas hot health spot. A landowner named Francis Wootan dug a well. The water tasted fine, but it turned everything washed in it a reddish yellow color. And those drinking it felt better. If they were ill, they got well. Wootan was so successful promoting his newfound healing water that he built a hotel to house the many visitors who came to drink and bathe in it. A bottling works was developed, a school was built, and soon people were coming from all over to imbibe and wallow in his miraculous well water.

Like Hughes Springs and Tioga, Wootan Wells flourished during the wonderful-water-healing era, but by the early twentieth century, it died as medical science evolved and the economy changed. During the heyday, though, Texas thrived with more medical springs than you could shake a stick at. Hardin County's famous Sour Lake waters were visited by Sam Houston, who came to bathe his wounds from the Battle of San Jacinto. Caldwell County's famous Sour Wells were reportedly savored by Davy Crockett. Teddy Roosevelt was reported to have bathed in San Antonio's hot sulfur wells. Douglas Fairbanks, J. P. Morgan, Tom Mix, and Clark Gable were said to have sampled Mineral Wells's crazy waters.

To name a few more, there was Hanna Springs in Lampasas, Stovall's hot wells in Jack County, Langford's bathhouse beside the Rio Grande in Big Bend country, Kingston hot springs in Presidio County, Dalton Springs in northeast Texas, and the sulfur springs swamps in and around the town of Ottine in Gonzales County. And the list goes on.

* * *

Sir John Franklin, a famous British explorer, in May 1845, left London, England in a bid to discover the elusive Northwest Passage. The ships, the *Terror* and the *Erebus*, were equipped with the most modern technological advancements of the day. Locomotive steam engines powered the ships. Their foods were carried in containers sealed using the most modern techniques of canning. The expedition sailed off to conquer the Arctic world . . . and was never heard from again.

In the 1850s, the graves of several crew members were discovered. From the best the relief expedition could tell, the men began dying within a year after setting sail, a peculiar finding since the expedition had been so well provisioned and planned.

In 1981, Canadian scientists discovered bones believed to belong to crew members of the *Terror* and *Erebus*. Spectrographic analysis confirmed they were indeed from those of the Franklin expedition. Analysis also showed that the bones contained extremely high levels of lead. Franklin and his crew died of lead poisoning from eating food stored in "modern" lead-containing cans.

If the most learned scholars of the time like Sir Franklin, Dr. McLean and his "Balderdash" colleagues, and James Lynch were blindsided by something so simple as lead in their food, bacteria on their hands, or lithium in their water, what are we, the educated of today, doing to ourselves that we just aren't aware of?

Were James Lynch and Dr. Kilmer really onto something? Is homeopathy really bunk? Is there some substance (like insulin or endorphins or estrogen or dopamine) in the body that has the miraculous capacity to repair us from within? Even in frontier times, millions of people wouldn't spend hard-earned money and precious time off to continually visit healing wells that didn't work. Can faith, or a "natural water cure," really heal by releasing some hidden humor, some secret liquid or entity into the body, on which the conditions and proportions of physical and mental health depend? Is there something like lead or lithium in our water, or food, or air that has the ability to heal us or cause cancer or heart disease? Makes you wonder just how ignorant we really are, don't it?

Oh, by the way, they've changed the theory again on how much pure water (water without any caffeine, etc.) you need to drink per day. Now they're saying that as long as you drink eight glasses of water, *in any form*—Cokes, tea, juice, beer—you won't get dehydrated. Think I'll just buy beer from now on. Heck, it ain't that much more expensive than water, anyway.

Just as many of the frontier dosage forms, old remedies, and medical procedures have been swept away by the winds of time, so have the many famous hotels, bathing pavilions, and mineral-rich wells.

A young pharmacist friend who listened with interest as I read parts of this book to him, asked, "Wayne? For Gods' sake, where on earth did you learn about all these places like Tioga Wells and Hughes Springs?"

I smiled and replied, "Well, let's see. I cut my teeth on Gene Autry. He and Roy Rogers were my heroes when I was growing up. I already knew Tioga was Autry's home. As for Hughes Springs?" I went on, "Hell, son, that's where I grew up."

He stared off a moment, and then said, "Who was Roy Rogers?"

That young recent graduate, doctor of pharmacy, had never heard of a pill-silvering canister, a cachet, or a sugartit, either.

*Lord, forgive us our indiscretions, and protect us from our own ignorance.* (45–accessed September 5, 2002; 46–accessed September 6, 2002)

## ABRAHAM'S BLUE PILLS

Abraham had a vision and heard voices. For days he suffered from insomnia, tremors, and attacks of anger. His friends say he lived in a cave of gloom; his melancholy was the frequent topic of their discussions. He was often overheard talking to himself or someone—God, maybe.

At a meeting, he fell into a fit of fury, his face distorted, his actions lurid and majestic; terrifying in his wrath, out of the blue he caught a man by the collar, lifted and shook him until his teeth rattled. For fear he would take the poor man's head off, his friends broke his grip and pushed him away. Abraham went home, and when the sun went down that night, he fell into a deep sleep as fear and terror fell over him.

These outbursts of rage and bizarre behavior were not those of biblical Abraham. They were the ferocious fits of President Abraham Lincoln, flare-ups incited by a little blue pill he took in 1858 for depression.

In early 2001, a study published in *Perspectives in Biology and Medicine* shows that a common antidepressant known as "blue mass" pills could explain Lincoln's known neurological symptoms.

Robert G. Feldman, M.D., an expert on heavy metal poisonings at Boston University School of Medicine, and Ian Greaves, M.D., an associate dean at the University of Minnesota School of Public Health, coauthored the paper, the main purpose of which was to determine how toxic the pills were.

Blue mass pills, a staple of the period for hypochondriasis, better known as melancholy, were well documented as having been taken by President Lincoln.

Feldman and Greaves used a nineteenth-century prescription to formulate exact replicas of the blue mass pills. Compounding them in the same crude manner as was appropriate for the time, the pills contained mercury, honey, rose water, licorice root, and rose petals. They were analyzed, and it was found that each contained the equivalent of 375 micrograms of the solid mercury. The safe daily dose of any form of mercury is 21 micrograms. Two or three of the president's blue mass pills delivered well over eight thousand times the amount deemed safe by today's Environmental Protection Agency (EPA) standards. In short, President Lincoln, steady-at-the-helm, mature, and calm leader of our nation, was poisoning himself with mercury. After he jerked his opponent's head nearly off at the 1858 Lincoln–Douglas debate and had to be pulled from him, Abe went home. Having realized the pills were his problem, he never took them again.

President Lincoln was deemed the epitome of self-control. His calmness in the face of hardship and danger are well remembered. Had he not stopped taking those little blue pills when he did, the outcome of the Civil War and the future of our nation might have taken a different turn. (50–accessed September 6, 2002)

## THE SNAKE OIL LEGACIES

The most popular images of frontier medicines were the snake oil preparations. Peddled at medicine shows from the backs of wagons, the "drummers" were well known to stretch their claims a bit. The "entrepreneur hawkers" of the day used any number of tricks to sell their products. Traveling in shows and employing men to herald their arrival, they entered townships with circuslike fanfare. Lectures, skits, marching bands, and assistants who moved among the crowd helped lend moral respectability to their deceptive presence. Indians were frequently recruited to promote the "natural philosophy" of the remedies. In actuality, most of the old formulas contained no real snake oil at all. Many if not all were mostly alcohol and vegetable bitters that were sold on the strength of testimonials and the frenzy of excitement created by the medicine show itself.

A famous cowboy named Clark Stanley sold a snake oil liniment he claimed contained the real thing. He reportedly got slaughtered snakes from his home back in Abilene, Texas, and processed the "juices" into the product he sold nationwide from his plant based in New England. But since the ingredients in medicines were not required by law to be placed on the label, there was no way a trusting consumer really knew what was in the remedies. Anything that could cure rheumatism, neuralgia, sciatica, lame back, lumbago, sprains, toothache, frostbites, sore throats, and animal bites had to be a bargain at fifty cents a bottle. After all, Clark Stanley himself

*Medicinal iron was prepared from the purest iron available in frontier times—horseshoe nails and fence wire. The nails and wire were cut into small segments, placed in water to dissolve, dried into a fine red powder, and made into tonics and pills.*

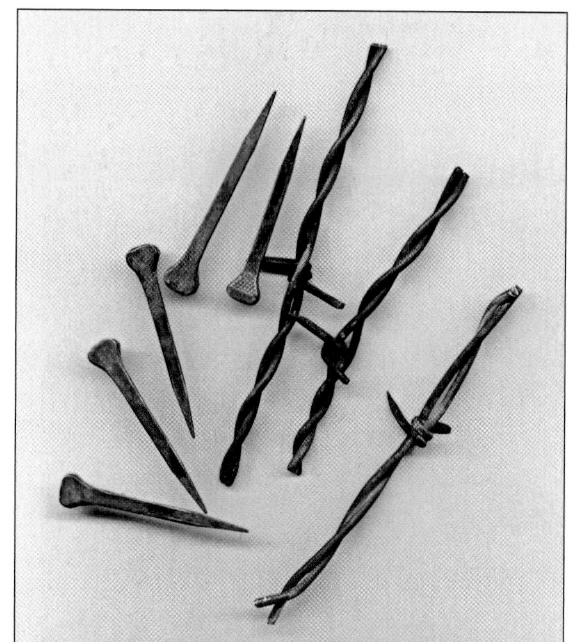

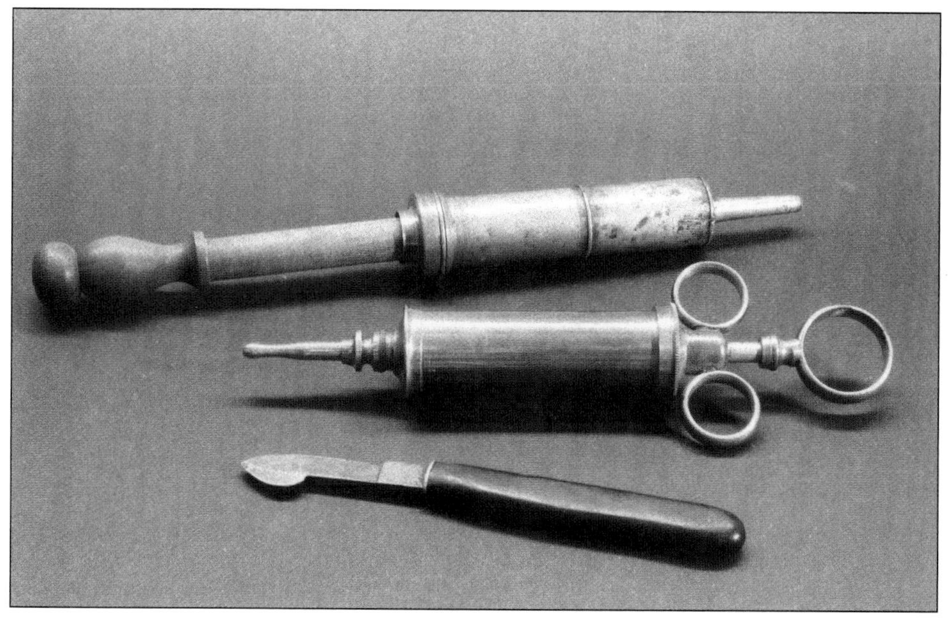

*A similar clyster syringe* (TOP) *was carried on the Lewis and Clark expedition. Clysters were used to administer enemas. Uro-irrigation syringes* (MIDDLE—*also called penis syringes) were used to flush the urinary tract with mercury solutions to treat venereal diseases. Bloodletting knives* (BOTTOM) *were used to bleed patients, the theory being to drain the body of the poison doing it harm.*

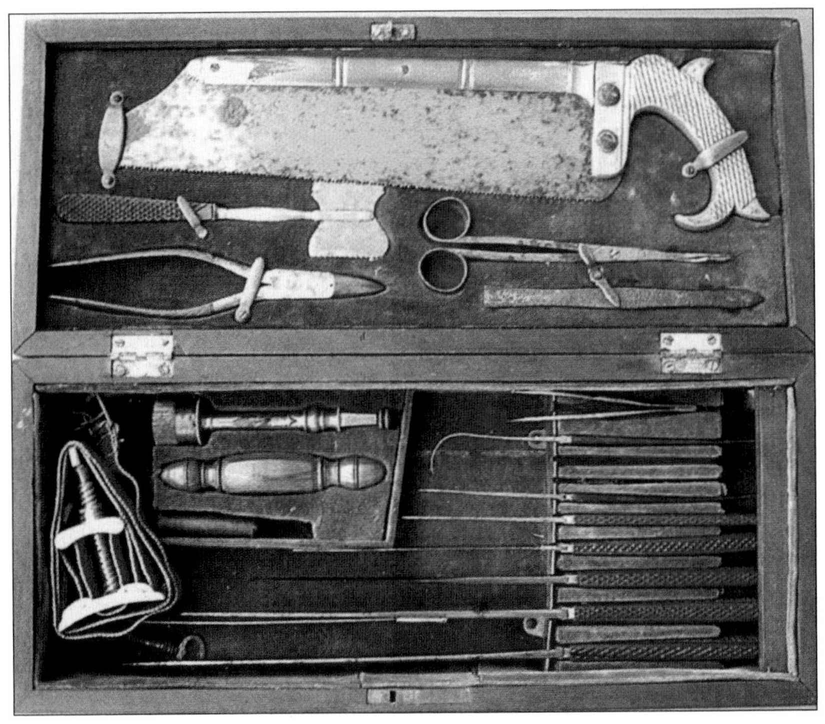

*Surgery during the eighteenth century was performed using gruesome tools of the trade. Note the bone saw* (TOP) *and the long probes* (BOTTOM) *used to "feel for" and remove bullets and arrowheads.*

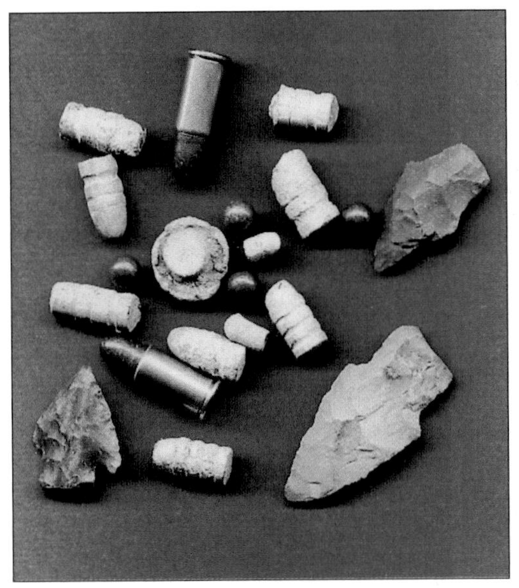

*Mushroomed bullets, musket balls, and arrowheads like those shown here were common items removed from bodies during pioneer times.*

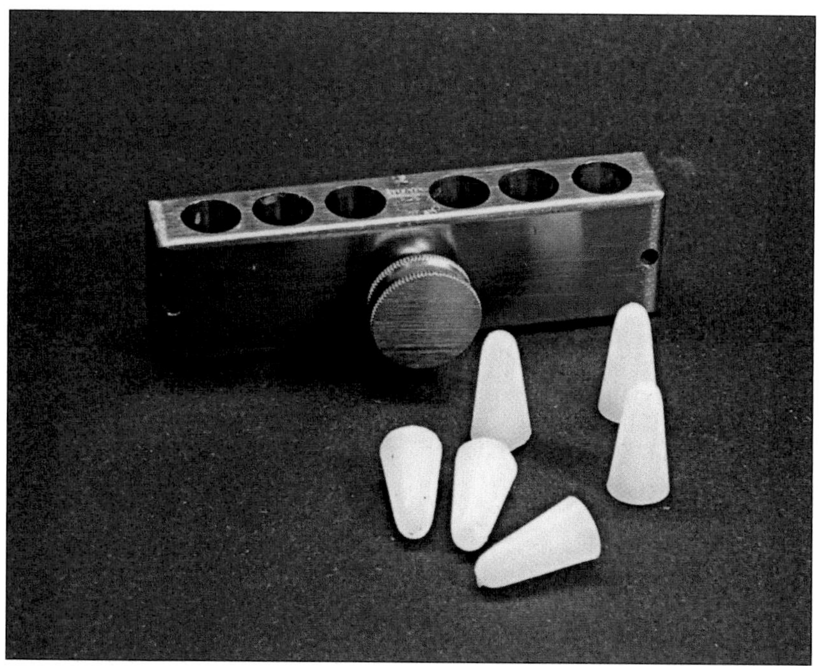

*Special molds, like the eighteenth-century one above, that bolted together were used to make suppositories. Cocoa butter and hog lard were used as bases. If the base was heated too hot, the active drug settled to the tip, sometimes making them layered looking and crumbly on the end—truly torpedo-tipped inserts, so to speak.*

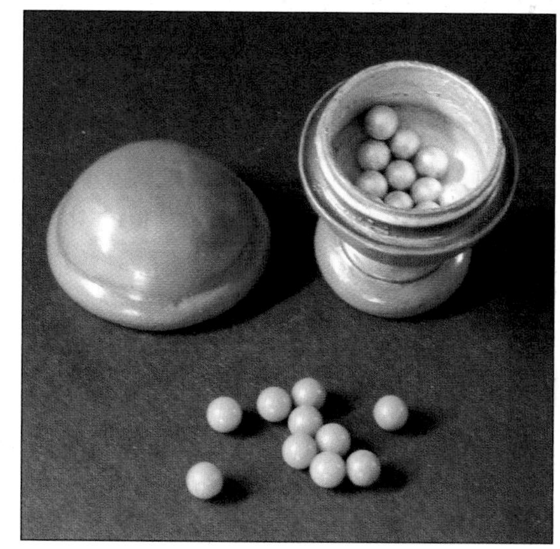

*Pill silvering canisters were portable, handheld devices used to coat pills after they were formed. Pills of the period were coated with everything from simple syrup to mercury or gold or silver.*

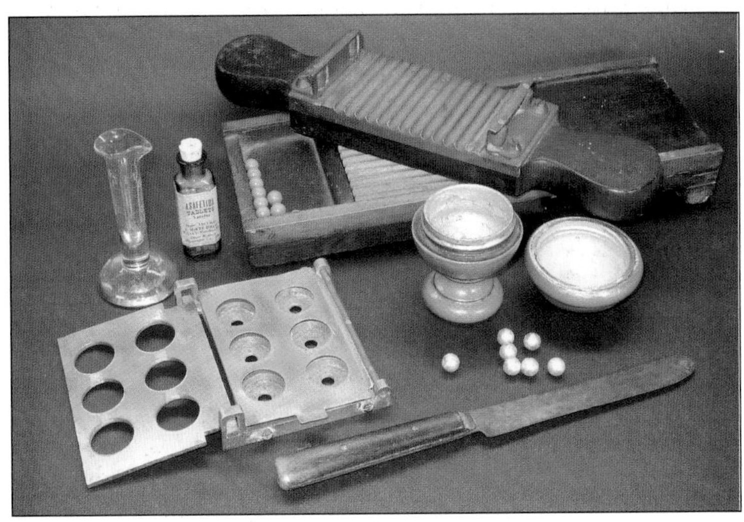

*Pill slides, or pill rollers* (TOP), *were used by druggists to form medications into uniform doses. Cachet machines* (BOTTOM LEFT) *were used to prepare oyster-cracker-like powder-filled dosage forms that were precursors to modern capsules. Note the long knife* (BOTTOM RIGHT) *used to cut and shape the doughlike materials.*

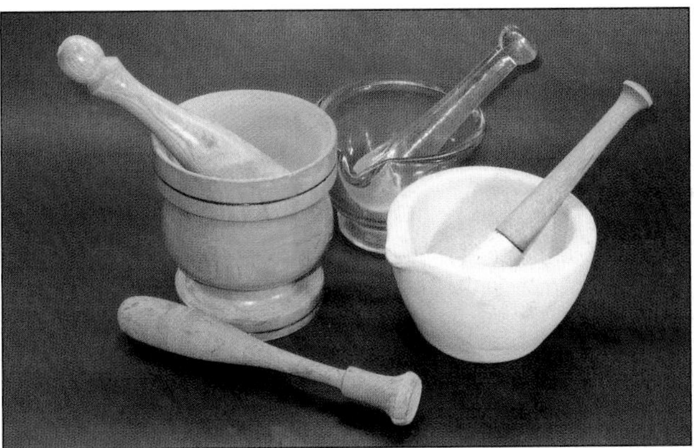

*Mortars (the bowl) and pestles (the handheld grinder) were used to prepare medications. Wood mortars and pestles* (TOP LEFT) *were used to grind lightweight herbs and plants. Note the wooden "clump buster" pestle* (BOTTOM LEFT) *with a concave end, which was used to break up lumps in powders and dried herbs. Glass mortars and pestles* (TOP RIGHT) *were used to triturate and mix fine powders into liquid bases. Porcelain mortar and pestles* (BOTTOM RIGHT; *note wood handle), were used to grind molten metal into chalk to flake it.*

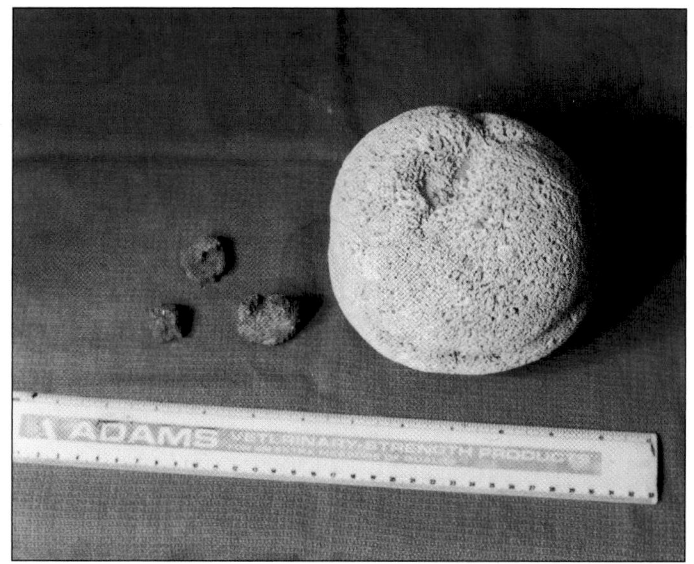


*Madstones like the above were obtained from animals, on the left are pieces of a single urolith (obtained from the bladder of a horse). On the right is a monstrous fecalith (obtained from the gastrointestinal tract of a horse).*

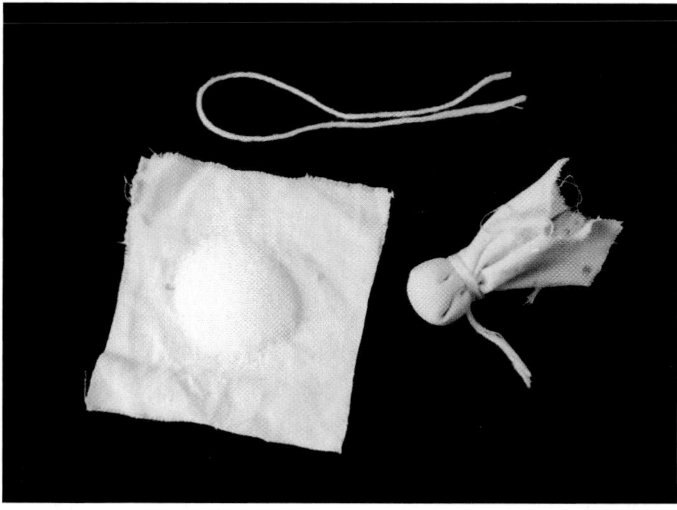

*Sugartits were used to administer doses of medication to babies. Sugar was placed in the center of a thin cloth and tied into a ball. The tit was then either dipped in drug or it was applied in drops and placed in the baby's mouth. As the baby sucked, the sugar dissolved and released the medicine.*

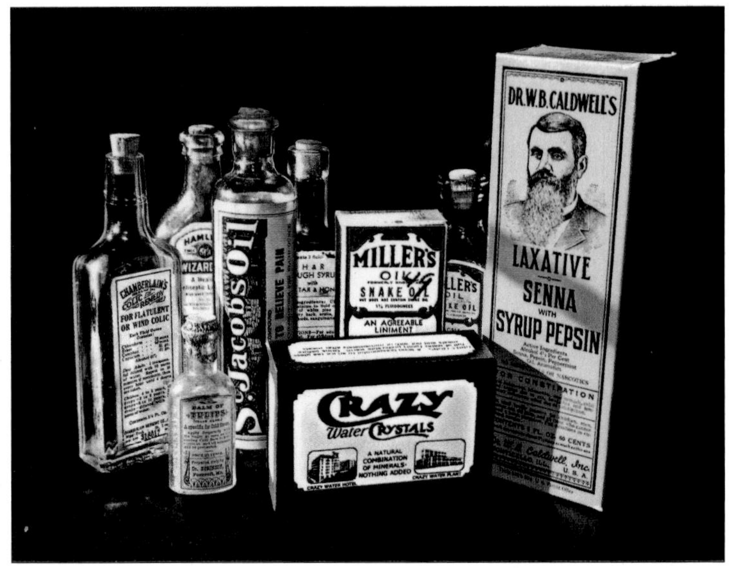


*Typical patent medicines available during the nineteenth and early twentieth centuries.* CLOCKWISE FROM LEFT, *Chamberlain's wind colic remedy, Hamlin's Wizard Oil, St. Jacob's Oil, H & R Coal Tar and Honey cough syrup, Miller's Snake Oil, Dr. Caldwell's Senna Laxative, Crazy Water Crystals, and the tiny bottle, Balm of Tulips.*

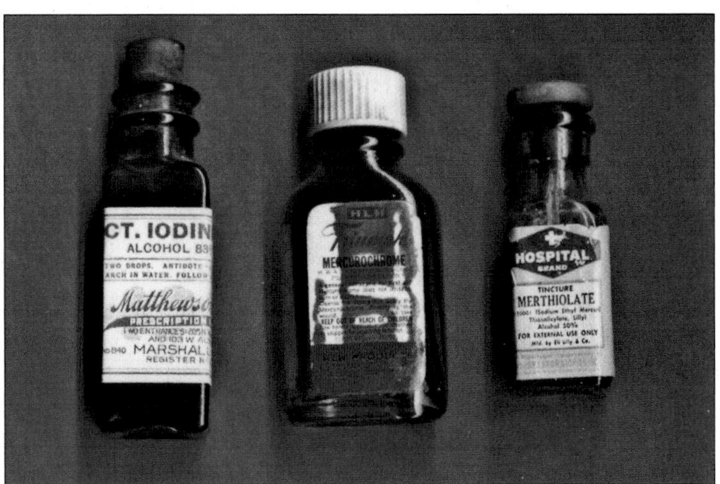


*The monkeybloods—tincture of iodine* (LEFT), *mercurochrome* (MIDDLE), *and merthiolate* (RIGHT). *All three were red badges of courage for cuts and abrasions.*

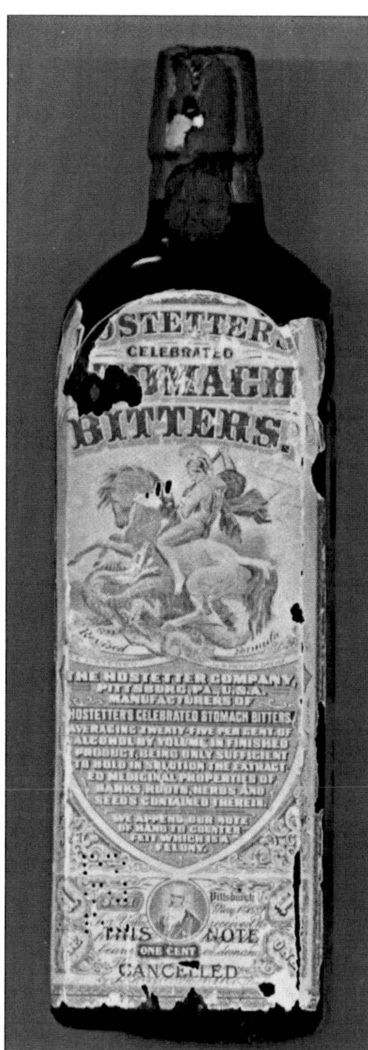


During the Civil War, Dr. J. Hostetter made millions off his stomach bitters. Boxcar loads of the "cure-all" were shipped to Union soldiers. With 44.3 percent alcohol, it's easy to see why the soldiers liked it.

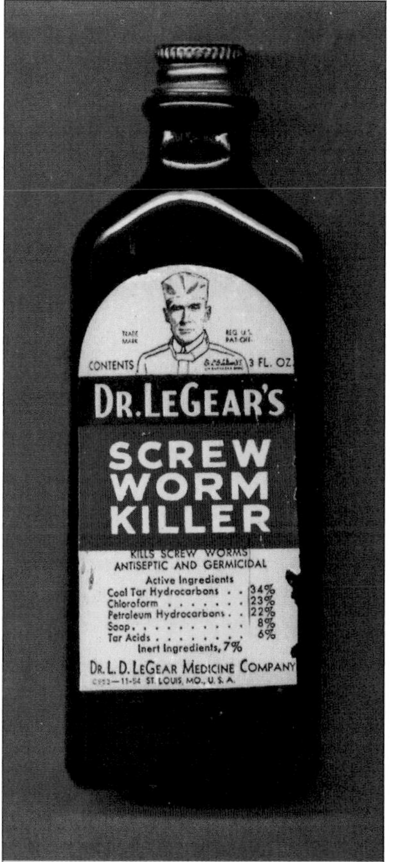


Screw worms plagued many a cowboy and farmer during frontier times. Dr. L. D. LeGear made his fortune off his formula. LeGear's antiseptic was used by humans as much as on livestock. Note the formula contains coal tar, which is still used and prescribed by skin specialists.

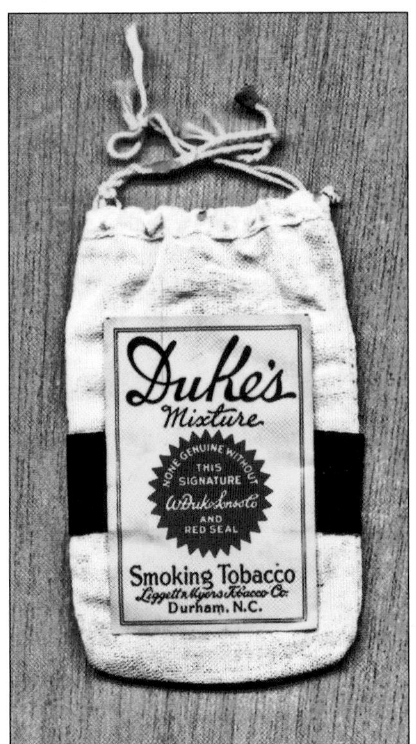


*Good old Duke's Mixture was a favorite of many a cowboy. Each bag came with a pack of rolling papers attached to the back. The smell of Duke's burning is a fragrant scent, like fresh pipe tobacco and fresh coffee brewing. Made even a nonsmoker desire a puff.*

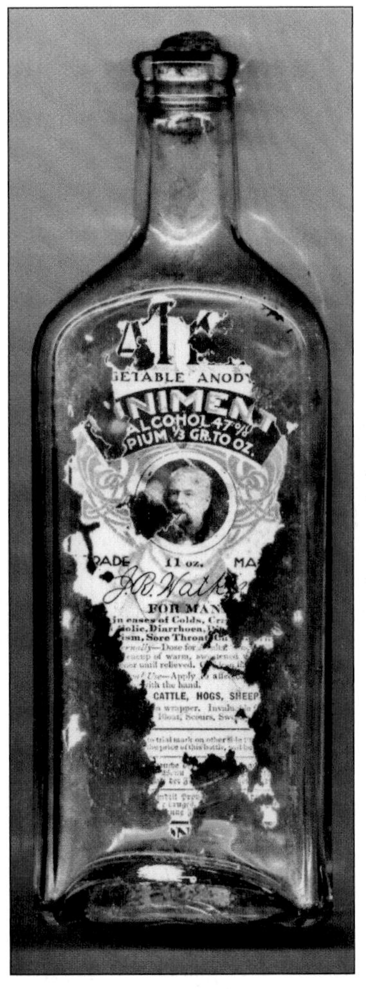


*Vegetable anodynes (painkillers) like Dr. Watkins Liniment pictured here claimed to heal everything from stopped up stovepipes to hogs with the runs. With 47 percent alcohol (that's 94 proof, folks) and third of a grain of opium to the ounce, is it no wonder the stuff sold? You plumb didn't care if you hurt or not.*

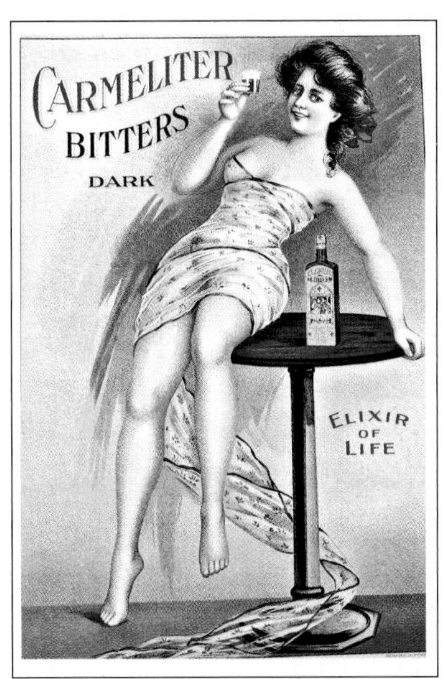
CARMELITER
BITTERS
DARK
ELIXIR
OF
LIFE

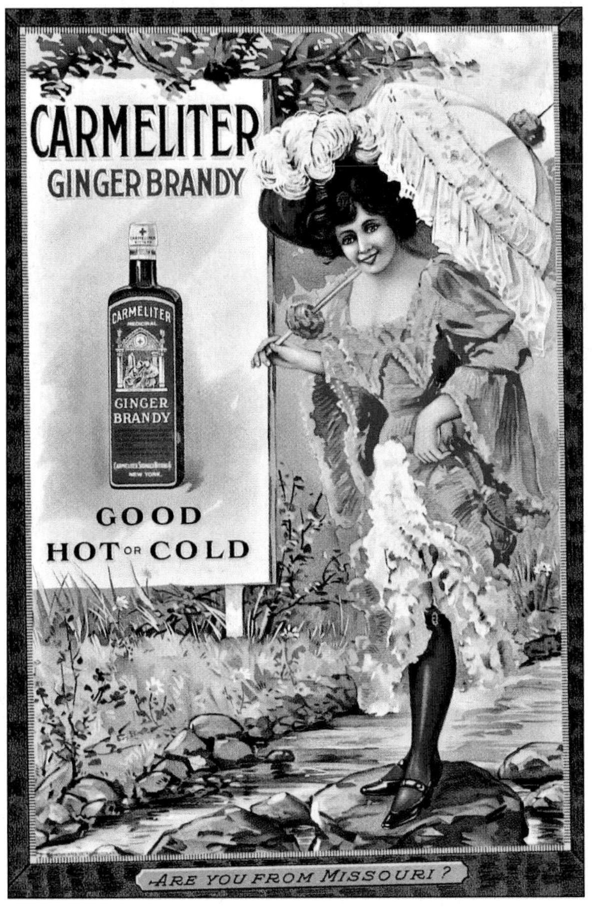
CARMELITER
GINGER BRANDY
CARMELITER
GINGER
BRANDY
NEW YORK.
GOOD
HOT OR COLD
ARE YOU FROM MISSOURI?

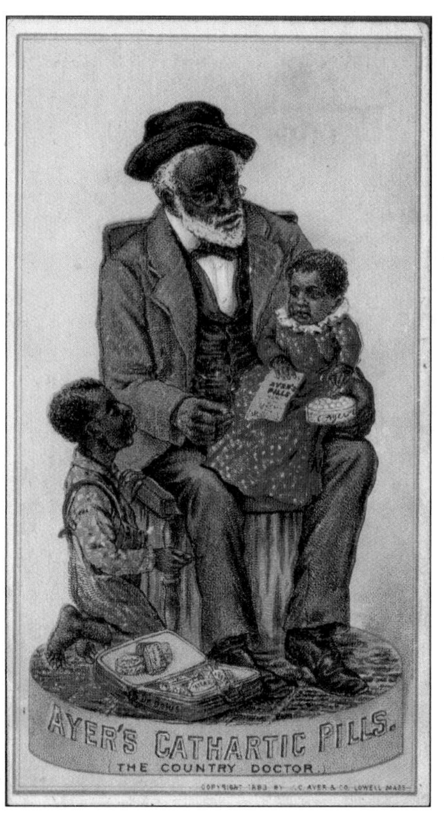
AYER'S CATHARTIC PILLS.
(THE COUNTRY DOCTOR)

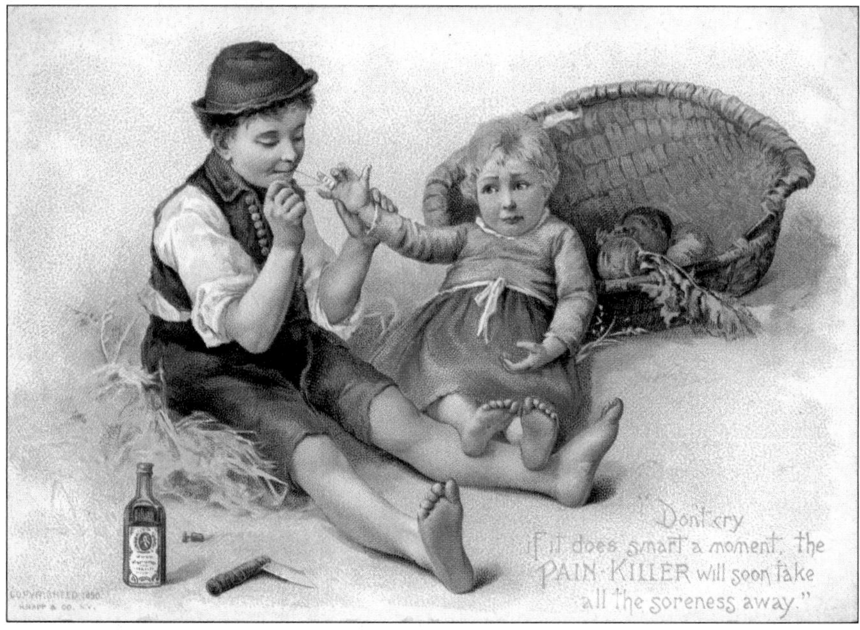
"Don't cry
if it does smart a moment, the
PAIN-KILLER will soon take
all the soreness away."

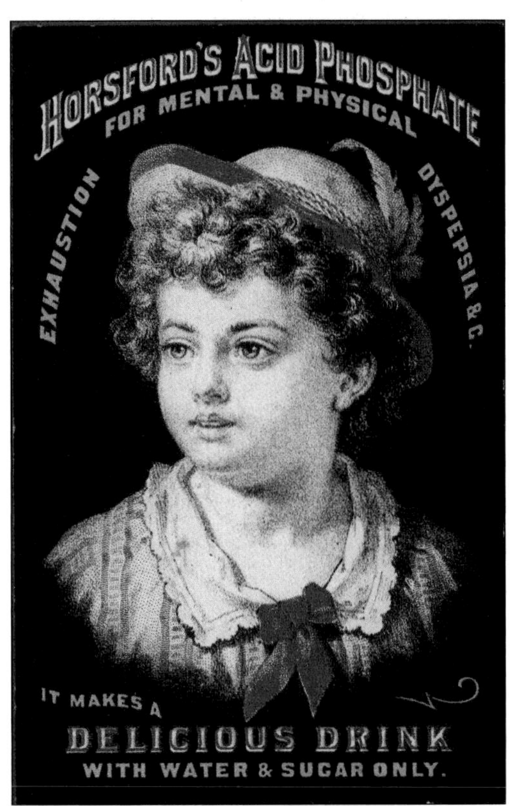
HORSFORD'S ACID PHOSPHATE
FOR MENTAL & PHYSICAL
EXHAUSTION
DYSPEPSIA &C.
IT MAKES A
DELICIOUS DRINK
WITH WATER & SUGAR ONLY.

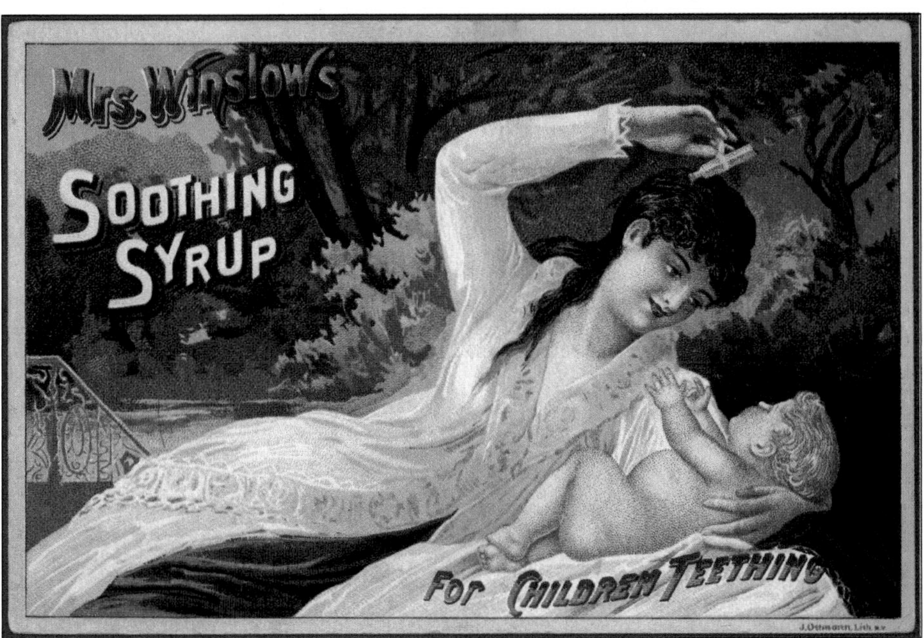
Mrs. Winslow's
SOOTHING
SYRUP
For CHILDREN TEETHING

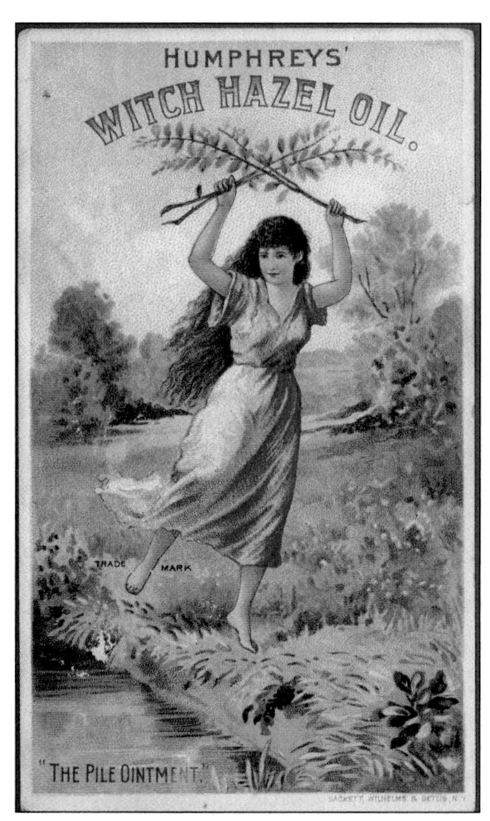
HUMPHREYS'
WITCH HAZEL OIL.
TRADE MARK
"THE PILE OINTMENT."

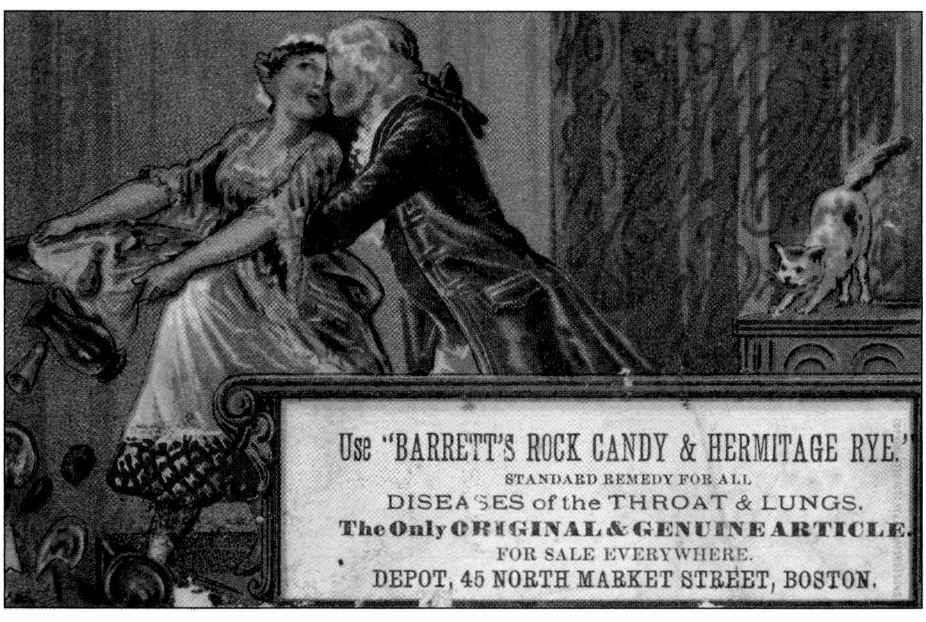
Use "BARRETT'S ROCK CANDY & HERMITAGE RYE."
STANDARD REMEDY FOR ALL
DISEASES of the THROAT & LUNGS.
The Only ORIGINAL & GENUINE ARTICLE.
FOR SALE EVERYWHERE.
DEPOT, 45 NORTH MARKET STREET, BOSTON.

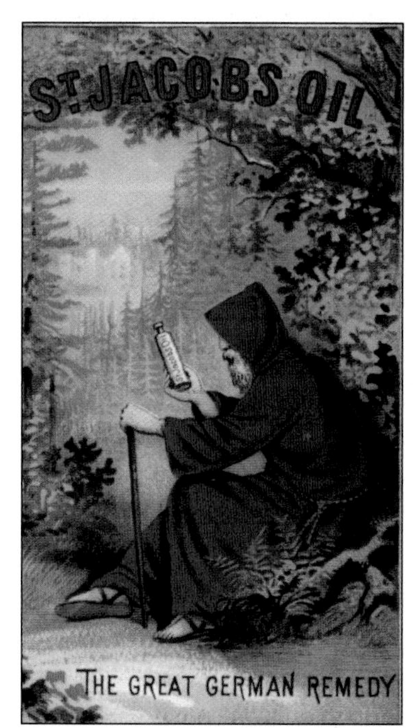
St. JACOBS OIL
THE GREAT GERMAN REMEDY

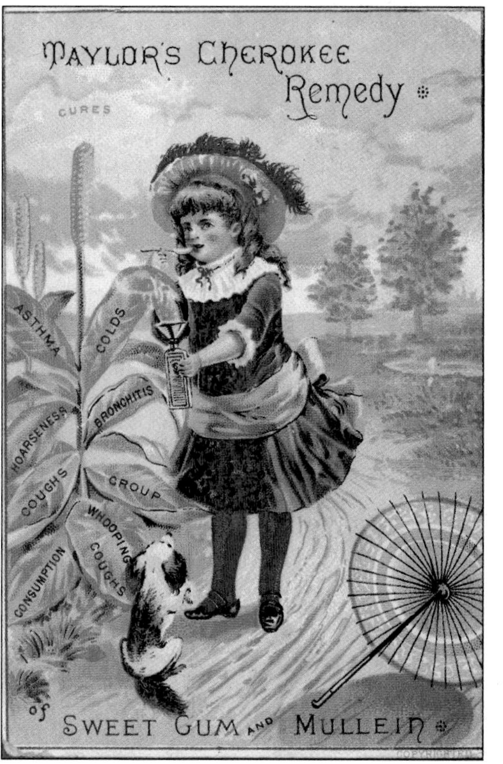
TAYLOR'S CHEROKEE
Remedy
CURES
ASTHMA
COLDS
BRONCHITIS
HOARSENESS
COUGHS
CROUP
WHOOPING COUGHS
CONSUMPTION
OF
SWEET GUM AND MULLEIN

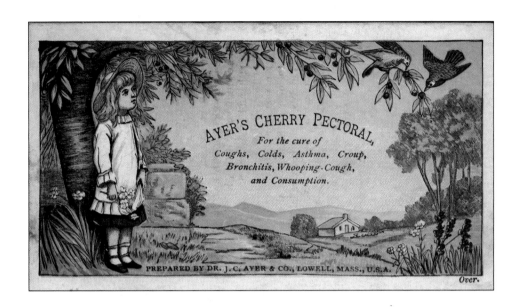
AYER'S CHERRY PECTORAL,
For the cure of
Coughs, Colds, Asthma, Croup,
Bronchitis, Whooping-Cough,
and Consumption.
PREPARED BY DR. J. C. AYER & CO., LOWELL, MASS., U.S.A.
Over.

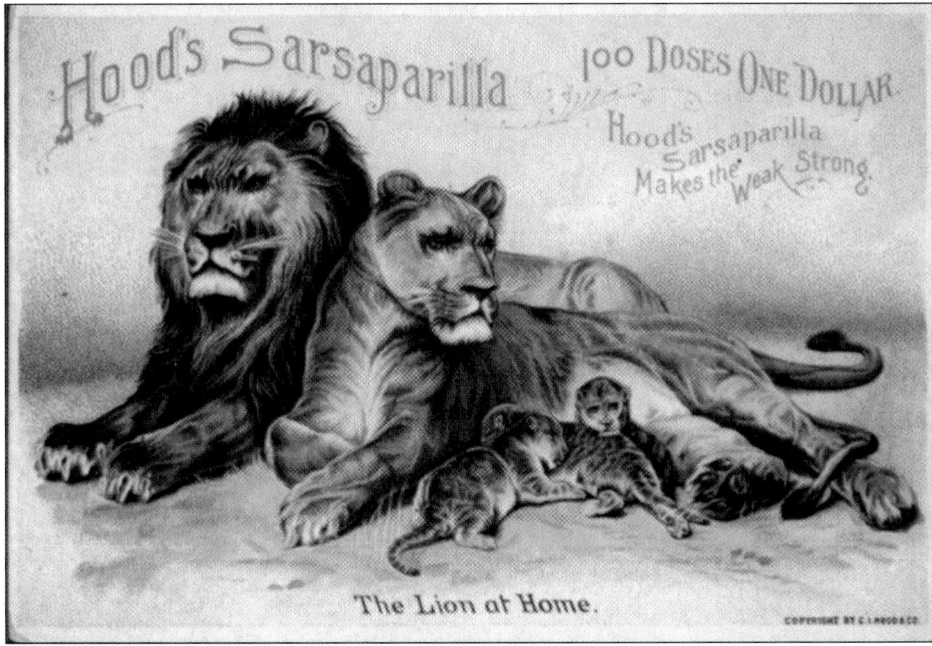
Hood's Sarsaparilla
100 DOSES ONE DOLLAR
Hood's Sarsaparilla Makes the Weak Strong.
The Lion at Home.

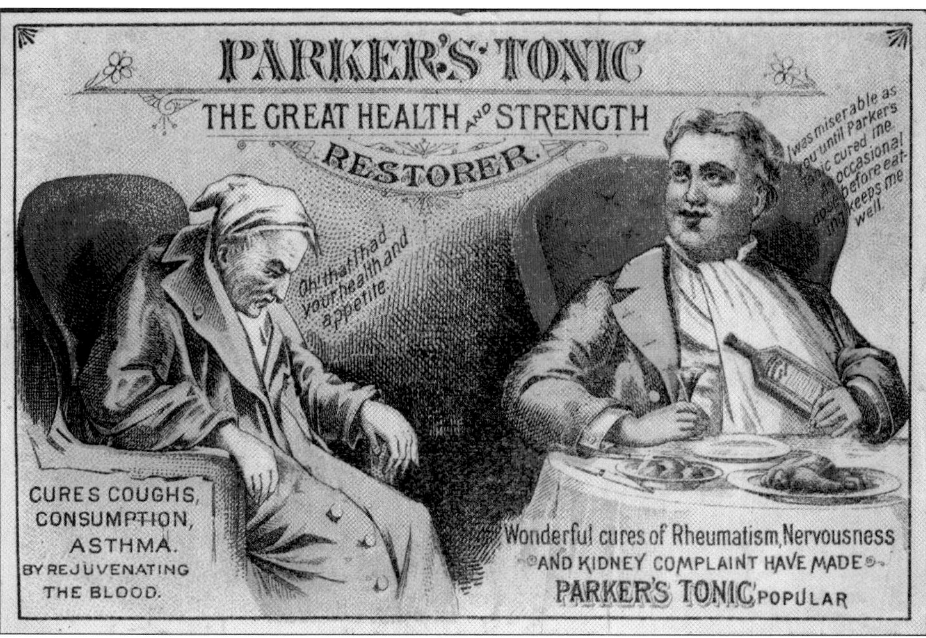
PARKER'S TONIC
THE GREAT HEALTH AND STRENGTH
RESTORER.
Oh! that I had your health and appetite.
I was miserable as
you until Parker's
ic cured me.
occasional
dose before eat-
ing keeps me
well.
CURES COUGHS,
CONSUMPTION,
ASTHMA.
BY REJUVENATING
THE BLOOD.
Wonderful cures of Rheumatism, Nervousness
AND KIDNEY COMPLAINT HAVE MADE
PARKER'S TONIC POPULAR

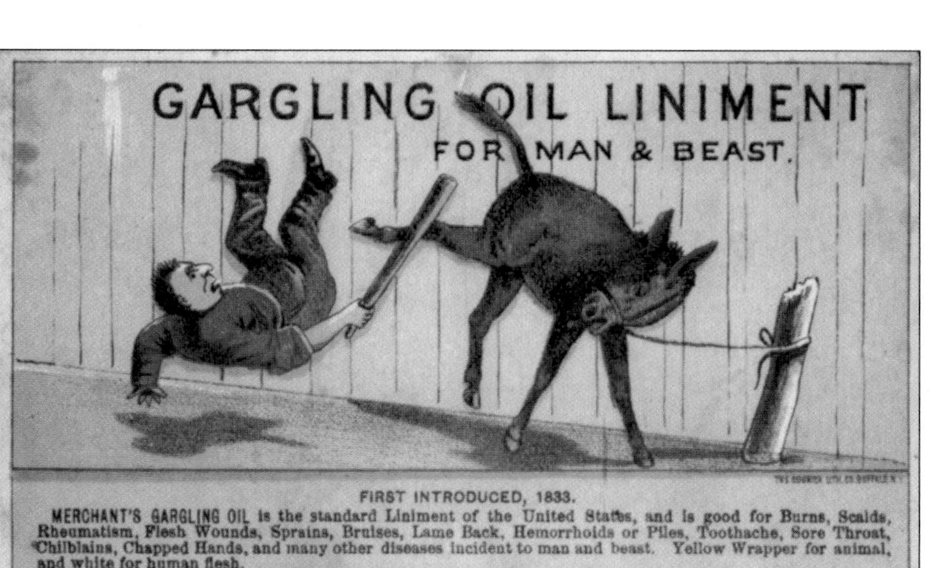
GARGLING OIL LINIMENT
FOR MAN & BEAST.
FIRST INTRODUCED, 1833.
MERCHANT'S GARGLING OIL is the standard Liniment of the United States, and is good for Burns, Scalds, Rheumatism, Flesh Wounds, Sprains, Bruises, Lame Back, Hemorrhoids or Piles, Toothache, Sore Throat, Chilblains, Chapped Hands, and many other diseases incident to man and beast. Yellow Wrapper for animal, and white for human flesh.
Manufactured at Lockport, N. Y., by M. G. O. Co., and sold by all druggists.
OVER.
JOHN HODGE, Sec'y.

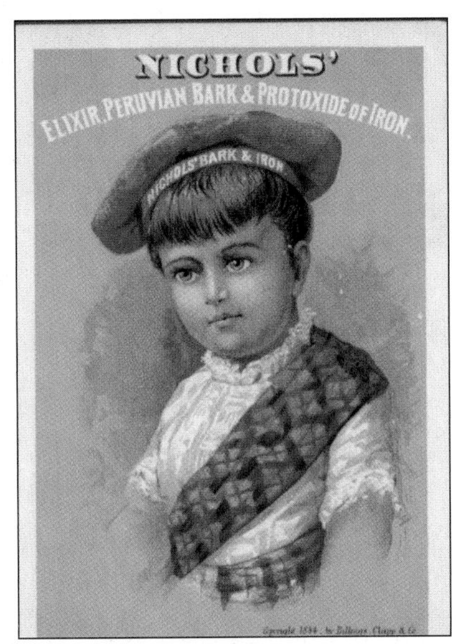
NICHOLS'
ELIXIR, PERUVIAN BARK & PROTOXIDE OF IRON.
NICHOLS' BARK & IRON

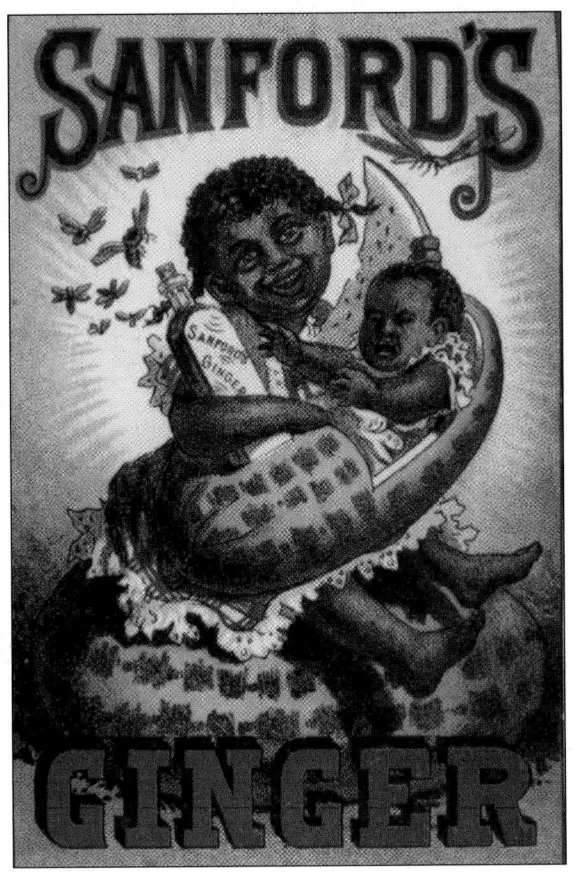
SANFORD'S
SANFORD'S
GINGER
GINGER

MILLER'S OIL

KNOWN FOR YEARS AS

MILLER'S

**SNAKE OIL**

BUT DOES NOT CONTAIN SNAKE OIL

Sold to and recommended by the public from coast to coast for more than fifty years. "Ask your neighbor about Miller's Snake Oil."

Recommended in the treatment of Minor Cuts, Burns, Bruises, Sprains, Insect Bites, Athletes Foot, Tired Aching Feet and Limbs, Sore Muscles due to exposure or exertion.

In cases of Minor Cuts, Burns, Insect Bites, pat the Oil onto affected parts gently.

Bruises, Sprains, Athletes Foot, Sore Muscles, Aching Feet and Limbs, bathe affected parts in warm water, or dry hot towel. Apply the Oil, rubbing gently over the surface.

Do Not Bandage

Satisfactory Results Guaranteed

For Horses and Cattle this Liniment is unexcelled.
PRICE 50c, $1.00, at all Druggists or by mail.

CAUTION: Discontinue use if excessive irritation of the skin develops. Avoid getting into the eyes or on mucous membranes

WE BELIEVE SNAKE OIL TO BE THE BEST PREPARATION ON THE MARKET FOR THE MONEY AND WE ARE CONFIDENT EVERY USER WILL BE DELIGHTED WITH THE RESULTS OBTAINED.

WE GUARANTEE SATISFACTION

**We list some remarks from thousands of letters of satisfied customers.**

I am writing to you about the Great Liniment made by your company, it gets results. Los Angels, Calif.

I think it is the best liniment I have ever used. Mason City, Illinois

I have used your liniment for years, it is the best I have ever had. Pamona, Calif.

Your Snake Oil is wonderful. Drexel Hill, Pa.

I have tried your Snake Oil and find it very effective. Everett, Wash.

My Brother gave me a bottle of your Snake Oil, I find it very good. Enderline, N. Dak.

I have tried your Snake Oil and think it is wonderful, I get great relief from it. Lost Creek, W. Va.

I have been using Snake Oil for a number of years and think it is wonderful. Milwaukee, Wisc.

I can't keep house without Snake Oil. Los Angeles, Calif.

Please send a bottle of Snake Oil as it is the only thing that does my Mother-in-law any good. Tampa, Fla.

We have used your Snake Oil for over 25 years. Brush, Colo.

Millions of bottles of Snake Oil have been sold during the fifty years and most of our sales have resulted from customers like you that have made recommendations to their friends or neighbors to try Snake Oil for various ailments. If you have found the relief you expected, tell your friends and neighbors about Snake Oil and the results you are getting. "Remember", for more than fifty years we have guaranteed that every purchaser of Snake Oil will get satisfactory results or your money refunded. We guarantee that regardless of price Snake Oil will give you more relief than any other product on the market.

Manufactured Only By

HERB PRODUCTS MEDICINE COMPANY

111 TUCKER ST. — JACKSON, TENNESSEE

BREWER PRINTING CO., JACKSON

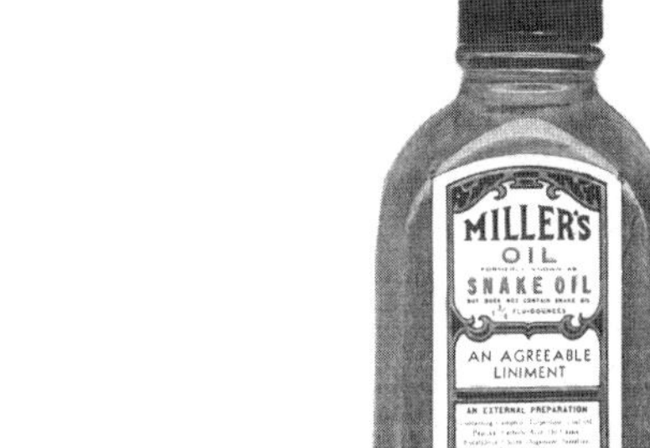

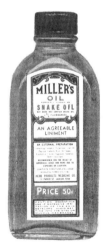

said this was the same recipe the Indians back home rendered from rattlesnakes and used to treat aching muscles and sore bones.

In 1917, the federal government seized a shipment of Stanley's liniment and found it contained little more than beef fat, kerosene, traces of red pepper, turpentine, and camphor, nary a drop of real diamondback rattler juice. Clark's quackery, over time, led *snake oil* to become synonymous with "useless cure-all."

Miller's snake oil formula, a popular remedy during the late nineteenth and early twentieth centuries, rode the tail winds of snake oil's reputation. Millions of bottles were sold, which contained camphor, turpentine, coal oil, paprika, carbolic acid, oil of cassia, eucalyptus, cloves, origanium, sassafras, and methylsalicylate, and they honestly said so right on the label.

The irony is, some of the old topical formulas actually worked on superficial aches and pains. As for their ability to "cure" such things as consumption and frostbites, well, that was a different story.

The American west has always been notorious for its outlaws. In nineteenth-century medicine, the country held true to its reputation. One of the most popular hawkers of all time was the famous "Doctor Lone Star," a.k.a. Texas Charlie Bigelow, a Bee County farmer who traveled the nation selling his potions and lotions, just like Clark Stanley did, in a carnival-style atmosphere. For one thin dime, his twenty or so road shows that stopped in rural areas provided entertainment in the way of animal trick shows, minstrel skits, singing, and dancing, all with the underlying purpose of selling his Kickapoo Medicines. Often, Doctor Lone Star and his partner, Doc. John E. Healy, planted shills in the audience who bought a bottle, sampled it, and with much ado proclaimed himself cured right then and there. One of their ploys was to have an agent selling the remedies in the middle of a crowd call out, "All sold out, Doctor." This precipitated a frenzied rush toward the other salesperson who still had bottles left in his hands. The out-of-stock agent would then rush for the stage and return with a few more bottles.

Healy and Bigelow's colorful characters ballyhooed their chopped grass (herbs) with shills (crooks) to squeeze (defraud) the country yokels (suckers) out of their hard-earned money. Television and radio today mimic the two doctors' gimmick of interrupting a good show to sell a product.

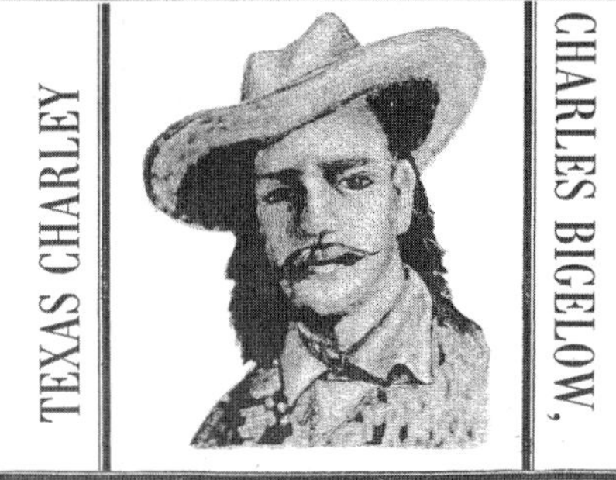
TEXAS CHARLEY
CHARLES BIGELOW,
GENUINE
KICKAPOO
INDIAN SAGWA
THE GREAT INDIAN MEDICINE
Is a compound of the virtue of Roots, Herbs, Barks, Gums and Leaves used for generations as Blood-making, Blood-cleansing and life- sustaining.
It is the Purest, Safest, and Most Effectual Cathartic Medicine known to the public.
WILL CURE
Constipation, Liver Complaint, Dyspepsia Indigestion, Loss of Appetite, Scrofula, Rheumatism, Chills and Fever Or any Disease Arriving from an Impure Blood or Deranged Liver.
FOR SALE BY ALL DRUGGISTS
PRICE $1.00 PER BOTTLE.

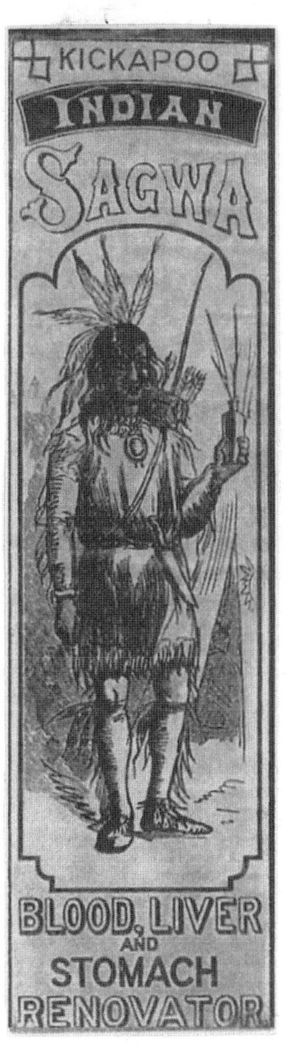
KICKAPOO
INDIAN
SAGWA
BLOOD, LIVER
AND
STOMACH
RENOVATOR

This Texas Therapeutic Road Show of Bigelow's reached its zenith sometime after 1880. Bigelow and Healy were the first to hitch the noble Indian to the medicine wagon. In 1881, they organized the Kickapoo Indian Medicine Company where hundreds of Indians were hired for atmosphere. The earliest of all Wild West shows was a come-on for Kickapoo Sagwa and other Healy and

Bigelow cure-all remedies. The famous Pawnee Bill was introduced to the medicine show business when he delivered a party of Pawnee Indians to Bigelow and Healy in Philadelphia when they were organizing their famous Kickapoo road shows.

Bigelow's partner, John Healy, was a shoe salesman who started out selling a magic vanishing cream door to door. After serving in the Civil War, he returned to New Haven where he made a batch of pain liniment he called King of Pain. With his profits from the liniment's sales, he organized Healy's Minstrels. There were no true blacks in his show. His Irish Thespians wore green velvets and billycocks and sang Irish ballads. While Healy traveled the country, in Baltimore, a Doctor E. H. Flagg concocted and sold a liniment from street corners, where he played a violin and sang.

Meanwhile, in Bee County, Texas, a lowly-born farmer named Charley Bigelow, whose only horsemanship involved a plow, was swapping his neighbors out of their possessions when he met a man by the name of Phil Grant, a.k.a. Doctor Yellowstone, who was traveling across Texas selling herbal remedies. Charley jumped right on Grant's bandwagon, learned a magic skit, let his hair grow long, and became a traveling medicine man.

Another medicine man named Percy G. Williams, in New York, was developing two other cure-alls, a liver pad and an electric belt. His medicated pad was clamped over the pit of the stomach to "absorb" through the pores and make new a neglected liver: a therapeutic novelty of the time. His electric belt, a boon to impotency, was a rave success and was copied by many other companies. Williams created traveling vaudeville-style acts to sell his wares. His success caught John Healy's eye. Healy dropped his minstrel show, teamed up with Flagg, and organized units to advertise and sell their own liver pads and the liniments. Among the first hired was a banjo player named N. T. Oliver, stage name Nevada Ned, and Charley Bigelow, who took the stage under the name of Doctor Lone Star. This new group first hit the road in 1879 with three units, each with a wagon load of foggy-eyed Indians, three entertainers, and a supposed doctor. The Kickapoo Medicine Company thereby became the first traveling chain of medicine shows.

E. H. Flagg's relative, John Hamlin, used and sold the same liniment formula (now called Kickapoo Indian Oil) as Hamlin's Wizard Oil.

It seems like forever that I have searched out the ingredients of this old formula. But even a blind mule occasionally stumbles through an open gate. Recently, at an old drugstore in a nearby town, while working so the owner could accompany his daughter to have a baby, I ran across an old prescription logbook in a display case at the store. Lo and behold, there in the middle of the partially decomposed ledger was the never before known formula of this famous remedy. Feast your eyes on a first, folks:

**Hamlin's Wizard Oil**

*a.k.a. Pain Balm, Flagg's Oil, and Kickapoo Oil Liniment*

Rx camphor spirits: 1 ounce
Ammonia spirits: ½ ounce
Sassafras oil: ½ ounce
Clove oil: 2 drams
Chloroform: ½ ounce
Oil of turpentine: ½ ounce
Alcohol (whiskey): 5 ounces

For one familiar with the saga of Jesse James, the name Charlie Bigelow rings a bell of familiarity. Nowhere, though, could I find on record a connection between Texas Charlie Bigelow of medicine show fame and the Charlie Bigelow from Texas who looked like and was buried as Jesse James in 1882. Jesse James reportedly sang at his own funeral, the casket of which contained the body of a man named Texas Charlie Bigelow.

Reportedly, a man named Jesse James came to Granbury, Texas, about a week before he died. Records at the Hood County Courthouse show a Jessie Woodson James died on August 15, 1951, at the age of 107. This sounds trim and proper, but history has a weird way of changing itself, particularly since no one lives to ask what really happened and how. There was a recent study done on Jesse James that nullifies the claims of his attending his own funeral. Scientists exhumed what was left of Jesse's grave in Missouri, and from DNA testing of tissues from known living descendants, it was proven that the real Jesse James was indeed buried in 1882. Who, then, lies in the grave in Texas? Is it the "real" Texas Charlie Bigelow of Kickapoo Indian Oil fame?

William Radam was yet another quack medicine huckster. An Austin gardener who raised his own herbs, Radam exploited the public with a mixture that supposedly "cured" by exterminating germs the same way he "debugged" weeds in his garden. Himself a Prussian immigrant to America who suffered from a variety of ailments, Radam was in constant search of a miracle medicine. He used the same theories to develop his microbe annihilator as he did to develop substances that killed fungi, blight, and microbes on his garden plants. He tested his product on himself. It worked so well he decided to promote it to mankind. The public fell for it with fists full of dollars. His Microbe Killer made him rich. By 1890, he had a string of factories from coast to coast. In 1888, he built the famous Koppel building on 322 Congress Avenue, in Austin, Texas. He later moved his fortunes to New York, where he lived in a mansion overlooking Central Park. He died in a life of luxury in 1902. His body lies interred in the Oakwood Cemetery, in Austin, Texas.

Radam's famous Microbe Killer was analyzed and found to contain 99 percent water, a smidgen of red wine, and a dab of each hydrochloric and sulfuric acids, nothing more.

## THE PERRY DAVIS PAINKILLERS

No composition on frontier medicines would be complete without the inclusion of Perry Davis's painkiller. Mark Twain even mentions it in his writings. Davis was born in 1791 in Dartmouth,

Massachusetts. He came from a poor family. Disabled at an early age, he became a shoemaker. In 1828, he helped invent and design a better grain mill. Hard times and sickness overcame him at the age of 47. His illness settled in his chest and caused severe intestinal problems and other troublesome ailments. His search for personal relief put him on the path of healing herbs. He wasn't very optimistic about his progress until a certain combination of medicaments began to make him better. Near destitute but eager to promote his product, he sold his horse and wagon and assembled a batch of his painkiller at a market in Boston. In 1843, he took his preparation to a crowded fair in Pawtuxet. Here he set up his stand and offered his formula to the public. He was an instant success. By the next year, he had purchased a building and was manufacturing his medicine on a factory scale. During the Civil War, his factory was taken into custody by the United States government to make medicine for army horses and soldiers. His son, Edmund, joined him in business in 1850. Perry died in 1862. Edmund died in 1880 after passing on the company to his newly acquired partner, Horace Bloodgood. The Perry Davis & Son operation was moved to New York City in 1895.

Christian missionaries distributed Davis's wonderful vegetable painkiller across the nation and abroad. Interestingly enough, though the word *vegetable* appeared in ads and on containers, his product contained no vegetables. A trademark-registered product holder during Perry Davis's time wasn't required to expose the active ingredients to the public. His remedy was mostly alcohol and opiates—a commercialized form of plain old laudanum. (52–accessed September 12, 2002; 54–accessed September 12, 2002)

## DEAR LYDIA

Born in 1819 in the little town of Lynn, Massachusetts, Lydia Estes was a teacher, nurse, and one who opposed slavery with a passion. In 1843, she married Isaac Pinkham. Due to her husband's financial difficulties, to help make ends meet, she formulated and began marketing an herbal tonic she called Lydia E. Pinkham's Vegetable Compound. As sales gimmicks, she published pamphlets and wrote articles and began answering letters in magazines. In essence, Lydia E. Pinkham became the nation's first Dear Abby. Naturally, each of her replies included recommended doses of her vegetable compound to treat whatever ailed the troubled inquirer. Her factory hired all female employees who answered questions and prepared her nostrums. She expanded her line of products to include liver pills, a blood purifier, and a sanitary feminine wash. Her product line helped "cure" women of everything from anemia and rheumatism, to fallen wombs and tumors.

Her most popular potion, her vegetable compound, has undergone many changes through the years to comply with modern laws. But still today her compound contains essentially the same ingredients. Jamaican dogwood, pleurisy root, licorice, dandelion, gentian, motherwort, black cohosh, and 10 percent alcohol (solely as preservative and solvent they claim) are still in it, along with vitamin C and vitamin E to make it more modern. And it is still available through drugstores today.

Did or, rather, *does* her compound work? From an old ad comes this testimonial:

> Eight years ago, I got into an awful condition with what the doctor said was a falling womb. I would have spells of bearing down pains until he would give me morphine, and when I could not stand that, they would put hot cloths to me. The doctor said I would never have children without an operation. A neighbor, who knew what your medicine would do, allowed me to give Lydia E. Pinkham's Vegetable Compound a trial. I did so and I have never had a return of my old trouble. The next September I gave birth to as healthy a boy as you can find, and now I have two more children.

Had this claim been a singular testimony, doubt as to the product's usefulness would have reigned supreme, but there are literally thousands upon thousands of similar claims on record that tout the success of Lydia's old formula. So, the next time you or someone you know gets a fallen womb, now you at least know what frontier women did for it. (62–accessed September 6, 2002; 63–accessed September 6, 2002)

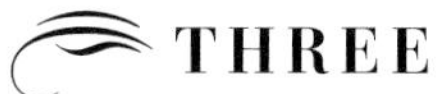 THREE

# *Frontier and Pioneer Drugs: A Folk* Materia Medica

THE GREEK PHYSICIAN DIOSCORIDES, in 78 B.C., described in his *De Materia Medica* thousands of plants that had medicinal properties. A surprising number are still important today: opium, ergot, hyoscyamus, and cinnamon. In 23–70 A.D., Pliny the Elder compiled thirty-seven volumes employed as references for many years. The Greek pharmacist/physician Galen (131–200 A.D.) devoted considerable time to assembling knowledge of how to prepare medicines, which he distributed in some twenty books. It was from Galen's humble beginning that pharmacy and medicine gradually went their separate ways, with the physician diagnosing and prescribing treatments, and the pharmacist or apothecary (the drug specialist) collecting, storing, and preparing the remedies. The term *materia medica* became synonymous with medicinal materials and products derived from natural sources. Today physicians still practice medicine and pharmacists still practice drugs.

Until 1817, European pharmacopoeias were relied on as authoritative references for U.S. medical practitioners. In January of that same year, Dr. Lyman Spalding submitted to the New York Medical community a proposal for a standardized U.S. national compendium. Out of Dr. Spalding's efforts, several committees were formed, and in 1820, the first edition of *The United Pharmacopoeia* was published. Many dates for the following monographs are based on that first and subsequent *Pharmacopoeia*. Keeping in mind that drugs underwent proving periods before being inducted into any official issue, these "official" dates are often erroneous for historians or writers trying to tell a story or relate whether a drug listed here was in use during a certain period of early American history.

This section is a folk *Materia Medica* of sorts, a listing of drugs and treatments used by our ancestors. The times included are based on those periods before the development of modern medicine.

*Frontier times* refers to the period from the middle of the eighteenth century through the last three decades of the twentieth century. References to *pioneer times* are to the period after America's declaration of independence, through the middle of the nineteenth century and until the coming of the railroads.

## ACONITE (1762–1960)

Also known as monkshood, aconite is the dried tuberous root of the plant *Aconitum napellus*, family Ranunculaceae, a turniplike plant, a perennial herb of which there are several dozen species. Most aconite during the late pioneer and early frontier periods was grown in Spain and shipped to the United States. In minute amounts, it was used orally as a cardiac and nerve calmer. Applied topically, usually in tinctures and liniments, it was used as an analgesic. The Chinese used it, as did ancient Indians, as a poison on arrow tips and as a "death drink" for condemned criminals. The ground root tubercles, the most poisonous part of the plant, were used in early wars to poison an enemy's water supply. Medically, aconite was a common ingredient in rubs and liniments used to treat the pain of rheumatism, lumbago, neuralgia, sciatica, and arthritis and in dental poultices. Aconite was an ingredient in a very popular German-made remedy known as St. Jacob's oil, which was sold across early America that contained aconite, ether, turpentine, red coloring, alcohol, and water. Ads for this old remedy were found in newspapers throughout the country.

Chinese immigrants boiled the plant's leaves like poke salad, poured it off several times to remove the toxins, and ate it. The common oral dose of the standardized aconite root was sixty milligrams. (1–p. 363)

## ALUM (1750 TO DATE)

Alum is the crystalline, double sulfate of aluminum and potassium. A colorless, odorless powder, sweetishly bitter to taste, it was readily soluble in water. Most supplies were quarried and imported from China. Externally it was used as an astringent by adding a teaspoonful to a quart of warm water. Applied dry, it was used to remove "proud" flesh (an exuberant mass or fungus granulations, as in an ulcer) and as a styptic and an axillary deodorant. Chinese immigrants used it as a laundry additive to give the clothes a clean, fresh scent. Many old eyewash remedies contained small amounts of alum. Gargled, it soothed a sore throat. Taken internally, it appeased whooping cough, allayed internal hemorrhages and excessive sweating, and acted as an emetic for croup. It was prepared and dosed by placing a half a dram of the powder in a large glass of warm water and taken.

## ANGOSTURA (1824 TO DATE)

The bark of *Galipea officinalis*, family Rutaceae, also known as casparia, was usually prepared in the form of a bitter tonic to treat malaria, diarrhea, and as a stomachic. Large doses were cathartic and had emetic properties. Angostura bitters were quite popular during frontier times. Their main *medicinal* action was due to the alkaloids cusparine and galipine, which had antispasmodic properties. But perhaps its best-selling point was that it contained not 30 percent alcohol as most rotgut whiskies sold during frontier times but a whopping 45 percent alcohol—that's 90 proof, folks. Talk about an antispasmodic; a few swigs of that bitter stuff and you didn't care whether you spasmed out or not. In large enough doses, it would indeed have emetic properties, the same properties we Texans refer to today as a "bowl-huggin' hangover." (4–pp. 67–68)

## ANISE OIL (1500 TO DATE)

Anise is prepared from the dried ripe fruit of *Pimpinella anisum*, family Umbelliferae, the main constituent of which was aromatic oil. Though largely used as a flavoring today in everything from candy to trotline bait, its use in frontier times was primarily as a medicine: topically to treat lice, scabies, and psoriasis; internally as a stimulant, for nausea and as a stomachic, a diuretic, a pectoral, a pediatric flatulent for colic, and a diaphoretic. Anise oil is high in iron and calcium, which defends it use in tonics. The active ingredients anethole, dianethole, and photoanethole are estrogenic. It also contains the blood-thinning constituents, umbelliprenine, bergapten, and scopoletin. So you see, it was, after all, a very good addition to old remedies that actually did some good. One claim made in a research source declares that it increased lactation, induced menstruation, increased libido, and was used to "alleviate the symptoms of male climacteric, which is the period of life after reproduction functions stop." What does that mean? Danged if I know.

The usual oral dose was ten to thirty grains of the bruised or powdered seeds in the form of a tea made by boiling two teaspoonfuls of the crude drug in a half-pint of water. Dose of the pure oil was 0.1 milliliter, or two to four drops, on sugartits or in juice. Anise is also the flavoring in Paregoric. (1–p. 235; 4–pp. 68–69; 66–accessed September 28, 2002)

## APPLE CIDER VINEGAR (3000 B.C. TO DATE)

Ancient Egyptians have long been recognized as the inventors of the vinegar prepared by fermenting apples. Apple cider vinegar does have antiseptic properties, and it was used in the days of old to disinfect wounds, relieve the pain of sunburn, and treat insect and snake bites. It was also used as a compress for black eyes and bruises.

D. C. Jarvis, M.D., in his book *Folk Medicine*, based a lot of his practice on the use of apple cider vinegar. His theory was that many medical problems were caused by an imbalance in bodily acids and that taking the vinegar with honey corrected many illnesses by allowing the body to heal faster. He goes into great depths to stress the mineral contents of both honey and apple cider vinegar. Time and again he stresses that no other vinegar, save for wine vinegar, which was used by the Italians, even comes close to the beneficial, antibacterial effects of taking fresh apple cider vinegar. He makes a rather astounding discovery when he states on page 68 of his book (which, by the way, became a best-seller in the late 1950s):

> I give this illustration, which I hope will not unduly disconcert the reader. To observe what happens to bacterial life when vinegar is used, get an angleworm from the garden and put it on a board or other hard surface where you may observe it. Now pour apple cider vinegar over it. First it writhes as though in pain. In a few seconds it becomes motionless. In a few seconds more, it turns white. The vinegar has caused loss of life in just those few seconds, for the worm is now dead. In the same way apple cider will destroy bacteria in your digestive tract.

"Writhes as though in pain." "Dead." Rather astounding observations, don't you think? And I didn't know worms were a form of bacteria. Don't you just love deductive reasoning? The best I can get from that experiment is: If you drink apple cider vinegar, you won't get angleworms.

Anyone who tastes a diluted solution of apple cider vinegar (a teaspoonful in a large glass of water) will get a hint of the taste of buttermilk. For cooking, mock buttermilk can be made by adding a teaspoonful of cider vinegar to a glass of sweet milk; after all, buttermilk is little more than a naturally fermented form of milk. My grandma loved buttermilk. I can't stand it. How do you know when it's spoiled?

In the good doctor's defense, the active ingredient in apple cider vinegar, acetic acid, is still used today as an antimicrobial eardrop. The product goes by the name Vosol Otic. (41–accessed September 1, 2002; 42)

## ARSENIC (3000 B.C.–1920)

Arsenic is an inorganic compound that was available in many crude forms; its use can be traced back to ancient Chinese cultures. During the eighteenth and nineteenth centuries, its introduction into Western medicines underwent rapid development and use. The two most commonly used as medicine were the trioxide and iodide salts. Their primary use was as alteratives and tonics. The usual dose was 0.002 to 0.005 milligrams (1/12 to 1/30th grain). Arsenic's toxicity became its downfall. Consumption of the drug was responsible for the old adage "If it don't cure you, it'll kill you." Tragically, that was more truth than fiction. Its use as a folk remedy alterative has prompted its revival. Arsenic trioxide (injectable) is being experimented with today (with apparent success) to treat a type of leukemia (cancer of the blood cells) called acute promyelocytic leukemia (APL) under the brand name Trisenox. All other uses of arsenic as a drug have, for all practical purposes save for rat poison, been discontinued. (2–p. 64; 60–pp. 357–59)

## ASAFETIDA (1753–1960)

Also spelled *asafoetida* or called devil's dung, asafetida was a gum resin obtained from living roots of the plant *Ferula assafoetida*, family Umbellifarea. In Latin, *asa* means "gum," and *foetida* means "offensive in odor or ill smelling," and it did smell bad. Diluted or adulterated with glycerin or gypsum, asafetida was made into suspensions and used as a carminative for colic and as a stomachic. The adult dose was formally listed as four hundred milligrams—that's just a little bit over two pinches. The concoctions stunk so bad that many adults and children refused a second dose. Taking milk of asafetida, also known as DeWee's carminative, was like drinking pure onion juice without the pepper effect. Voodoo practitioners wore sacks around their necks that contained asafetida. It not only warded off evil spirits; it warded off people. Here's an interesting "doubt it or don't." Asafetida is, or used to be, one of the secret ingredients in Worcestershire sauce. (1–p. 285)

## ASPIRIN (1897 TO DATE)

Aspirin (acetylsalicylic acid) is classified as a salicylate. Salicylate usage in medicine can be traced all the way back to the fourth century B.C. when the powdered extract from the bark of willow trees was used to treat pain. The parent salicylate, salicin, was successfully isolated from willow bark in 1829. Sodium salicylate, aspirin's chemical precursor, was isolated in 1875. Acetylsalicylic acid (aspirin) wasn't isolated until 1897 by Felix Hoffman, a German chemist working for a company named Bayer, who set out to concoct a sodium salicylate that was less irritating to the stomach. He succeeded by synthesizing acetylsalicylic acid, which became known as aspirin—the painkiller of choice still today for physicians around the world.

Precisely how aspirin worked wasn't uncovered until the 1970s when it was discovered that it inhibits a hormonal-like substance in the body called *prostaglandin*. Prostaglandin regulates certain pharmacodynamic bodily functions such as pain sensitivity, swelling, redness, fever, and the agglutination of blood platelets and blood vessel elasticity.

A good-quality willow bark (fifth century to date) will yield approximately 7 percent salicin. Twelve ounces (a large coffee mug full) of willow bark tea was made by adding 4.5 grams (approximately one teaspoonful) of pulverized willow bark to a gallon and a half (5,778 milliliters) of water and steeped. When cooled, one cup of tea roughly delivered the equivalent pain killing effect of one 325-milligram aspirin.

Combining aspirin with caffeine had a synergistic action on the aspirin. *Synergism* means that caffeine (when taken with aspirin) makes the aspirin stronger, particularly for headaches. And thus was born Excedrin!

In the late eighteenth century, cinchona bark was in short supply. Cheaper and more readily available substitutes were needed. Two alternatives, acetanilide (1886) and phenacetin (1897), both had advantages over quinine of having pain- and fever-reducing properties. In 1893, another medicine, paracetamol, was isolated, but little use of it was seen until early in the twentieth century when it was discovered that paracetemol was a metabolite of both phenacetin and acetanilide. Paracetamol is another name for acetaminophen, known to many if not to all as Tylenol. Phenacetin was the *P* in the old APC tablets that were sold as the Empirin compound. Today, Empirin solely contains aspirin.

Willow bark steeped with coffee made a crude version of frontier Excedrin tea. Today, the combination is still used, with the addition of acetaminophen (Tylenol), as the only over-the-counter product available that has a legal indication for migraine headaches—Excedrin Migraine. (19–p. 9; 55–accessed September 13, 2002)

## BAMBOO

Bamboo is a plant, *Arundinaria japonica*, family Poaceae. Aside from the hard and dried stalk being ground up, mixed into food, and used to kill enemies in early China, the plant supposedly had medicinal value. Juice from the young shoots was hardened into a kind of sugar and used by Chinese factions in the early days of the west to treat asthma, cough, and gallbladder disorders. (4–p. 95)

## BARBED WIRE AND HORSESHOE NAILS (1753 TO DATE)

Most medicinal compendia in the eighteenth century came to the United States from Europe and were the sole sources of reference until America's first pharmacopoeia came out in 1820. *The Edinburg New Dispensary*, written by Dr. William Lewis in London in 1753, and other British medical references were used as blueprints for the U.S. pharmacopoeias. In this volume, the good Dr. Lewis went into great detail to explain the preparation of consumable iron from metal filings and segmented pieces of fence wire. He stressed the importance of using pure iron and a clean file.

A magnet was passed over the filings found around the base of a blacksmith's anvil. The fine particles were then tapped through a sieve onto a magnet to separate the purer elements. This fine dust was placed in a mortar and covered with water. The red rust fluid formed was decanted, placed in an open container, and allowed to dry. The final product, referred to as ruft of iron, was then ground into an even finer powder.

Dr Lewis continually stressed that the purer the iron, the better. Brittle iron like that used in plows contained other metals to make them harder. Fence wire, another softer form of iron, was cut into small segments and dissolved in the same manner as iron filings.

Ruft iron was well known to cause stomach pain and a condition called "eructation." Eructation! Eructation! I love it. "Boy, your husband sure had a big eructation, didn't he?"

Actually, it only means belching. "Eructations" were due to stomach acid acting upon the iron and releasing gas. It wasn't learned until much later that very little of the pure iron (the ferric form) was broken down inside the stomach to be of any real therapeutic value. A less irritating, much more therapeutically active form of medicinal iron was prepared by placing the same iron filings or fence wire segments in sulfuric acid. The mixture was warmed and allowed to effervesce, then dried by evaporation to leave a fine powder of iron called *sulphas ferri*, or ferrous sulfate (1753 to date), which is better known today as iron sulfate.

Adding a solution of iron sulfate to carbonate of soda formed carbonate of iron, another early iron salt. The two reacted to form a sulfate of soda/carbonate of iron mixture called *black oxide of iron*. This iron carbonate was called *chalybeate* and was what made many of the old tonics black in color. Chalybeate was as irritating to the stomach as ruft iron and had to be taken in small doses throughout the day. The chalybeate springs of Hughes Springs, Texas, were naturally rich in iron carbonates.

Ferrous gluconate was a later addition to the less stomach-irritating irons. The gluconate and the ferrous sulfate forms of iron are the active ingredients in the modern products, Feosol and Fergon, which are for iron deficiency anemia. (10–pp. 64–67; 61–p. 444)

## BARLEY (1753 TO DATE)

*Hordeum distychum*, family Gramineae, aside from its use to make beer, when eaten or boiled into tealike infusions was used to treat bronchitis, diarrhea, stomach disorders, and generally to make you feel better. Its "feel better" action was in the beta-glucan it contained that slowed the stomach's emptying rate and helped stabilize blood sugar. An ointment prepared from hops, *Humulus lupulus*, of the mulberry family was another bitter plant used in making alcoholic beverages. During the latter part of the nineteenth century, hops was a very popular topical remedy for chapped skin.

Barley contains enzymes and hordenine, a sympathomimetic agent that stimulates blood circulation and dilates the bronchial tubes. The enzyme *diastase* is responsible for barley's fermenting ability.

*Diastase*? So that's what makes Scotch taste so good. Three cheers for diastase. (4–p. 95)

## BAT CRAP (GUANO)

Petrified bat crap was a natural source of potassium nitrate. Centuries-old bat dung heaps from caves solidified into a valuable frontier medical and military resource. *Nitre*, also known as *potassium nitrate* or American saltpeter (saltpeter) (1753 to date) was mixed into a paste with alum and applied to the hollow of decaying teeth to relieve pain. Nitre acted as a diuretic and diaphoretic to help cleanse the body, but it cleansed in other ways, too. Calvary soldiers and young men in institutional situations were slipped nitre into their food to soften their sexual urges. Extreme physical exhaustion, a probable reduction in bodily fluid volume, and night sweats lessened the men's desire to do anything but sleep. Mixed with sulfur and charcoal, nitre was also made into gunpowder. Farmers claimed it made an excellent fertilizer.

The usual oral dose of nitre was ten grains.

## BEESWAX (300 B.C. TO DATE)

Beeswax is the wax purified from honeycombs that was secreted into the cells by worker bees. After separating the honey, the comb is placed in hot water. Skimmed off and filtered, the melted wax was poured into molds and allowed to cool and harden. Beeswax varied depending on the locale from yellowish to gray-brown. It had an agreeable odor and sweet taste. Chinese immigrants took it orally for diarrhea, hiccoughs, and the relief of pain. It was primarily used as a malactic (an emollient to soften and soothe skin), as a vehicle for topical folk medicines, and as a thickening agent and fragrant, male-attractant base for earlier cosmetics. The old "Um, you smell good, like honey," is where Texans got to calling "honey" someone whom they liked, loved, or admired. (1–p. 195)

## BELLADONNA (1504 TO DATE)

Also known as deadly nightshade, devil's berries, and naughty man's cherries, Belladonna is the dried flowering tops, leaves, and fruits of *Atropa belladonna*, family Solanaceae, a perennial herb indigenous to Asia Minor and Europe. The drugs mydriatic (dilates the pupils) properties were first recorded in 1802. It wasn't until 1860 that its analgesic properties were recognized. Belladonna contains hyoscyamine, scopolamine, and atropine. Belladonna is a central nervous system stimulant, the effect of which is followed by depression. Its most useful property was its ability to decrease the flow of most bodily secretions: saliva and sweat. In crude tonics its primary sedative effect was on the gastrointestinal system whereby it slowed the movement of the intestines, bladder, and other internal organs. It was customarily made into tinctures that were given orally in less than one-milliliter doses up to three times daily. Orally, it was used for bronchial spasm, gut spasms, and whooping cough. Teas made from the plant's leaves were used by Italian women to give them a striking appearance by dilating their pupils. Supposedly, this made them appear more attractive, cordial, and relaxed. They were more cordial; they stumbled, couldn't see very well, and just sat around smiling.

A major problem with belladonna's preparation was that it was often adulterated with poke root. Belladonna's active ingredients, atropine and hyoscyamine, and their synthetic derivatives are still used today as antispasmodics and mydriatics. (1–p. 302; 4–pp. 103–4)

## BENZOIN (1300 TO DATE)

Also called almond tears and styrax, benzoin is a sweet-scented gum resin obtained from the plant *Styrax benzoin* and *Styrax paralleloneurus*, family Styraceae. Cutting the bark and allowing the sticky exudates to collect in containers attached to the trees is how it was obtained. The residue was formed into blocks and sold. Benzoresins contain cinnamic acids and resinotannols. Orally, it was

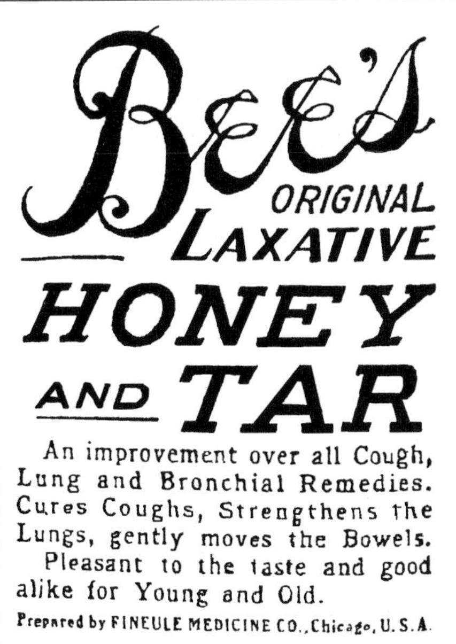


used as a stimulant, an expectorant with diuretic properties, and an inhalant for upper respiratory symptoms. Typically, a teaspoonful of benzoin tincture was added to a pint of hot water. A towel was soaked and wrung, held over the face, and inhaled. Topically it was used as an antiseptic and skin protectant on blisters that was often referred to as "tough skin." (1–p. 288; 4–p. 105)

## BEZOARS

Also known as *madstones*, or magical gut rocks, bezoars were rocklike formations that developed within the innards of ruminants (cows, horses, buffalo, deer, etc). Just as a grain of sand becomes embedded in an oyster to form a pearl, hair balls, small rocks, or dirt masses that were ingested while eating grasses, that or bits of metal or other foreign materials, calcified inside the stomachs of ruminants to produce gut rocks. As medicine, these stones were highly valued by frontiersmen. Anywhere from ten pounds to as small as a pea or a kidney bean, the stones were the accepted remedies for the bite of a mad skunk, fox, or dog—hence the name madstones. The stone was sometimes soaked in hot sweet milk and applied to the bites. Legend had it that the rock "sucked the pizened slobber right out." They were also applied to heal boils, festered cuts, inflamed bunions, bullet holes, snake bites, spider bites—anything that seriously needed the "pizen" drawn out of it.

In frontier days, madstones were considered priceless and were so cherished they were passed down from generation to generation. It wasn't uncommon to have someone show up at your cabin door to ask if they could use your crude pearl from a deer or buffalo's gut—your madstone—to cure a "black widder" bite or the like.

These gut rocks consisted primarily of magnesium, calcium, chromium, nickel, copper, and lead. Any small particulate object or quantity of hair eaten by a buffalo or deer or antelope could serve as a nidus (core) for the progressive layering of mineral deposits that formed the stones. Their incidence, due to the sheer magnitude of the massive herds, was greater during the time of the buffalo than it is today.

Bezoars were of several types and came in many sizes, shapes, and forms depending in which part of the animal's innards the rock formed, but even then, each one was unique in its own way. *Enteroliths* and *fecaliths* formed in the animal's stomachs, intestines, and colons. *Uroliths* formed in the bladders and urinary tracts, and *coleliths* formed in the gallbladders. The ones most used as madstones were the bladder stones, gallstones, and intestinal stones. Sometimes the stones grew large enough to close off the intestines and kill the animal, but most were found during field dressing or slaughtering. Some of these valuable stones were retrieved from hardened buffalo patties and other dried animal excrement. A smooth rock that had pimples, was porous, and had a corallike surface was likely a bezoar that the animal had passed.

The stone's crude absorptive properties were the mechanism for its "drawing" actions. Realistically, a large portion of people bitten by a rabid animal didn't get rabies, anyway. Trying to convince an old pioneer that the rock really didn't save his life was like trying to tell my grandma Leorah that "witching a well" had no scientific basis, either.

In pioneer times, superstition or not, owning a piece of the rock was its own form of insurance against sure misery and likely death. (64–p. 5, accessed September 23, 2002; 65–accessed September 23, 2002)

## BLACK PEPPER (1753 TO DATE)

*Piper nigram*, family Piperaceae, the source for black pepper, was the dried form of the plant's fruit. Aside from its use as a condiment, taken orally, it was used as a medicine to stimulate menstrual flow and as a diuretic, an antiflatulant (to reduce bowel gases), and a tonic. Black pepper contains piperine, which is a known abortifacient. Native Americans used Indian long pepper (*Piper longum*) for the same purposes settlers did black pepper. Red pepper and cayenne do not contain the active ingredient, piperine.

The hot peppers—red, chile, cayenne, and so forth—have been used for centuries as painkillers. Capsaicin, a natural chemical derived from these plants of the Solanaceae family, is still used today under the trade name of Zostrix. The mechanism of action of these hot pepper entities isn't fully understood. Evidence suggests that the chemicals in them prevent reaccumulation of Substance P (no, not urea) that renders nerves insensitive to pain. A more understandable explanation may lie in the drug's ability to alter endorphin levels. Endorphins are the body's natural painkillers. These are very powerful internal painkillers, much more powerful than even morphine. Some people get a "runner's high" from eating hot chile peppers. In some cultures there are reported pepper addicts. This makes sense. Hot peppers, like nicotine, alter the body's state of consciousness. Just as sustained exercise creates a kind of stress-pain on the central nervous system, the more pain, the more endorphins—the drugs in hot pepper does the same thing. Maintaining steady pain from the chemical constituents in hot peppers floods the brain with interruptive thought processes that overwhelm the senses with a sort of "rush." You need not worry about hurting yourself by eating too many hot peppers. Granted, they may burn going and "leaving," but they seldom if ever blister or cause any real damage.

Many hot peppers are available for the addicted pepper lover. One called *Capsicum annum* grows in Louisiana and Texas and matures to a fire engine red to illustrate its feverish content. The pepper is a thick, wrinkled curving pod with a rounded head and a cleft at the end. It is said to be hot enough to make your lips smoke. The devilish little fruit gets its name not from its fiery color at maturity but from its anthropomorphic, anatomical semblance to a part of the human body. The spicy outgrowth goes by the name peter pepper. If you are interested, seeds are available from any seed company that specializes in peppers. (4–p. 590; 34–accessed August 17, 2002)

## BONESET (88 B.C. TO DATE)

Also known as feverwort and Indian sage, boneset consisted of the ground, dried leaves and flowering tops of *Eupatorium perfoliatum*, family Compositae. The plant was indigenous to eastern and central North America. It was believed that boneset relieved breakbone fever, which was caused by a virus. North American Indians and colonists used it in the form of a strong tea to treat fever, indigestion, malaria, and snakebite, and as a diuretic and laxative. Boneset tea was made by placing a heaping teaspoonful of the ground-up plant in a pint of boiling water and allowing it to steep for ten to fifteen minutes. One cup of the tea was taken three times daily. A 1:1 fluidextract in 25 percent alcohol was dosed at two milliliters. A tincture made with 45 percent alcohol was dosed at half teaspoonful three times daily. (1–pp. 165–66; 4–p. 168; 56–accessed September 13, 2002)

## BORAX (10 A.D. TO DATE)

Boron, also called *Subboras sodae*, is one of 109 elements that make up our planet. Trace amounts of it are everywhere: in water, plants, and animals. Combined with oxygen, it forms boric acid (1702 to date). Atmospheric conditions, rain, and volcanic condensation redistribute the mineral all over the planet. It is found naturally in the borate state. One of Texas's earliest saddlebag doctors, John A. Veach of Jasper County, moved to California during the gold rush of 1849. On his way there he discovered massive borate deposits in the Mohave Desert. He moved on then to Oregon, where in 1870 he chaired the department of chemistry at Williamette University.

It wasn't until 1872 that Death Valley's borate deposits were mined. Twenty-mule team wagons were used to haul the rocky deposits, hence the name of the most famous Borax producer of all.

Boric acid was used for catarrh (inflammation of the nasal and mucous membranes with drainage). Combined with glycerin it was applied as an anti-inflammatory for skin irritations and was mixed

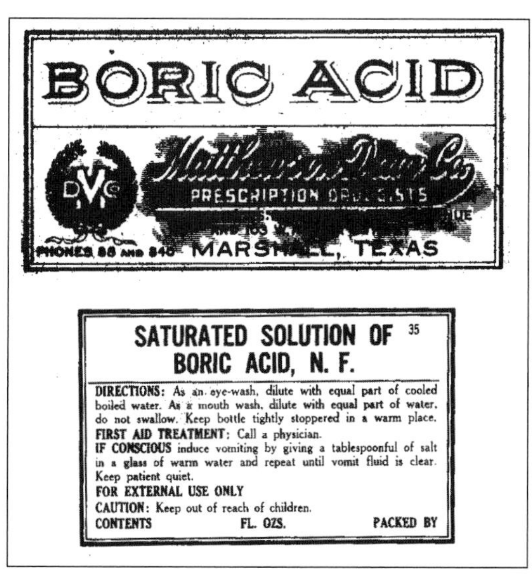

in shampoos. In a saturated solution, it was used as an eyewash and as a mouth rinse for inflamed gums. Though poison, borax, in small doses, was taken for headaches. It either cured or killed. It is still used today in roach poisons. (12–p. 183; 57–accessed September 13, 2002; 58–accessed August 13, 2002)

## BUCHU (1842 TO DATE)

Buchu, also known as bucco, is the leaves and oils of the plants *Barosma betulina*, *B. crenulata*, and *B. serratifolia*, family Rutaceae. The oil from the buchu plant was often used as a flavoring agent. Diosophenol, a camphorlike chemical in the plant, is thought to be the active ingredient. Diosophenol's ability to irritate the kidney may define its diuretic activity. Much like pollen or a foreign object in the eye or on the nasal mucosa makes them water to eliminate it, buchu irritated the kidney and made urine flow. Frontiersmen used buchu for cystitis and prostatitis, and other genitourinary conditions, and as a carminative. It is also an abortifacient. A common dose was two grams of the dried leaves in a suitable liquid. Extractives of buchu leaves are still used today in Dr. Kilmer's Swamp Root Herbal Tonic.

## BUCKEYE (1753 TO DATE)

Also known as horse chestnut and Spanish chestnut, buckeye comes from the plant *Aesculus hippocastanum*, family Hippocastanaceae. The plant was native to Asia and northern Greece and North America. The seeds, leaves, and bark of the tree were used. Seed extracts were mostly used, which contain a saponin, aescin that promotes circulation and treats venous insufficiencies. The plant also contains sterols, flavonoids, and tannins. Topical preparations were used to treat hemorrhoids, sprains, and varicose veins.

A teaspoonful of the pulverized bark from the tree's branches

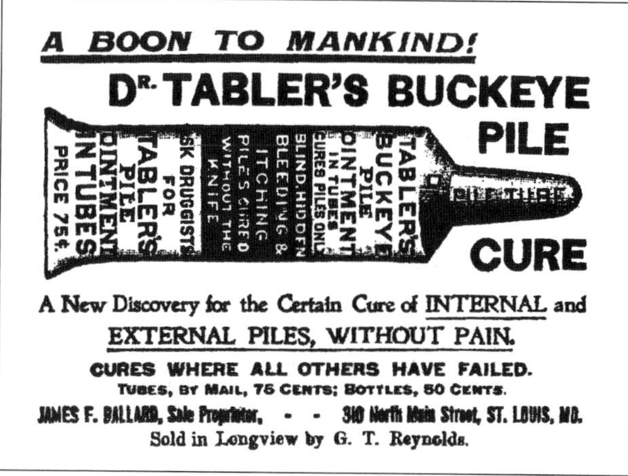


was steeped in a cup of water and taken for diarrhea and catarrh. The shells of the green seeds contain poisons and if taken orally in sufficient amounts could be lethal. Roasting the seeds is said to destroy its poison content. A popular remedy that Texans bought a butt-load of (pun intended) was Dr. Tabler's Buckeye Pile Cure. The ointment was said to "'cure" when all else failed. (59–accessed September 13, 2002)

## BURDOCK (1753 TO DATE)

Burdock, also known as cocklebur, is the dried first-year roots of the plant *Arctium lappa*, family Compositae. The dried and powdered roots were taken straight or imbibed in tea form. Many folk remedies contained burdock and were said to "purify the blood" and cure everything from head colds and acne, to cancer and a leaning chimney. Save for the chimney, they might have been right. Burdock extracts, which contain arctiopiricin, are active against both gram-positive and gram-negative bacteria. It has also been proven to have some antitumor and antimutagenic activity. (4–p. 190; 12–p. 204)

## CALAMINE (1740 TO DATE)

Also known as smithsonite, calamine (zinc carbonate) was a naturally occurring ore that contained silica (sand) and iron. Calamine was excavated, roasted, dried, and pulverized into a fine pink powder. Before the eighteenth century, the Romans made brass by mixing smithsonite ore with copper and heating the mixture. The heat was sufficient to reduce the ore to metallic state but not melt the copper. The vapor from the zinc permeated the copper to form brass, which could then be melted to give a uniform alloy. As a medicine, calamine was mixed into pastes and prepared in suspensions, which were applied to the skin as drying agents to help heal excoriations. Calamine's use became more popular after 1867 when phenol (carbolic acid) was discovered. A 1 percent phenol and calamine suspension was used for poison ivy and is still available today. No records of the internal use of calamine could be found. (10–p. 564; 61)

## CAMPHOR (1753 TO DATE)

Camphor was a ketone obtained from the evergreen tree *Cinnamomum camphora*, family Lauraceae. Indigenous to Asia, it was naturalized to the States. Crude camphor gum occurred as a crystalline exudates in the clefts in the wood of the stems and roots. It was prepared by steam distilling chips and sawdust of the tree. It was then purified by sublimation. Applied locally, camphor was used as a weak antiseptic and a mild anesthetic, antipruritic, and rubefacient. Taken internally with magnesia or charcoal, it acts as a stomachic for pyrosis. Camphor induces vasoconstriction of the nasal passages to give a decongestant effect. Dispersed in turpentine as a liniment, it was very popular as a soothing, cooling liniment for arthritis, aches, and pains. Camphor is the main ingredient in Campho-Phenique and many other commercial products used today. (60–p. 724)

## CARBOLIC ACID OR PHENOL (1867 TO DATE)

Phenols occur naturally as volatile oils and were prepared by the destructive distillation of plants such as *Thymus vulgaris* and *zygis*, family Labiata, to produce thymol; and *Eugenia caryophyllus*, family Myrtaceae, to produce eugenol. For many years, distilling crude coal tar, then separating and purifying the distillate by continued crystallization produced a purer more commercial form of carbolic acid. Phenol has a characteristic oily, sweet, and almost smothery petroleum odor. It was used as a caustic, disinfectant, and topical anesthetic. As a germicide, it is still the standard against which the antibacterial activities of modern antiseptics are compared. Common concentrations used were: in lotions for poison ivy and skin pain, 1 percent; in ointments for hemorrhoids and so forth, 2 percent. Five drops of a 5 percent mixture in glycerin, olive oil, turpentine, or coal oil (followed by a cotton plug) were used quite effectively for earache. (1–pp. 238–31; 60–p. 1262)

## CASCARA SAGRADA (1894 TO DATE)

Cascara sagrada is the dried bark of the buckhorn tree, *Rhamnus purshiana*, family Rhamnaceae. The medicinal was called "sacred bark" by the North American Indians. The bark was stripped during the summer beginning in May, sun dried with the outer bark exposed to the sun, and then stored for a year before using. Cascara contains anthraquinone glycosides, which the body breaks down to give its laxative and curative action. The bark was pulverized and made into bitters by adding alkaline clays (dirt) or magnesium oxide and fluid extracts. The common dose of the bitter extract was one milliliter (three hundred milligrams). It was often made in combinations with aromatic oils into a tastier aromatic preparation as a tea, which was easier to take. Adding two grams (a scant half-teaspoonful) to six ounces of boiling water and letting it steep for ten minutes, straining, and adding a few drops of peppermint or anise oil and a smidgen of sugar made a fairly pleasant-tasting concoction. Cascara was more than just another cathartic; it reportedly restored the bowel to a healthier tone, which made repeated doses unnecessary. In small doses, it was used for pyrosis and as a stomachic. (1–p. 113; 4–p. 232)

## CASTOR OIL (1800 TO DATE)

Castor oil was extracted from the beans of a bushlike tree indigenous to India, *Ricinus communis*. *Ricinus* is Latin for "tick"—the resemblance of the seed and their markings to the insect. The hulls of the seed are removed, and the hearts are compressed with huge rollers, which expel the oil.

When I was in pharmacy school, while working on that project on "Drugs Used on the Chisholm Trail," several other pharmacy students were on our committee. Castor oil was one medicine on my list for research. Anyway, we uncovered a passage in some records about an old Cajun woman who macerated spider legs, rattlesnake tails, and who knows what else, in castor oil and used the concoction to remove warts. If memory serves me right, she lived somewhere in Louisiana. Well, you had to know my buddy, Ken Ellis, who helped me do the research on this old woman. Ken was a prankster from the word go.

One day I dropped by his pharmacy in Marshall, Texas, to visit him. We hadn't seen each other in years. While we laughed and

**CASTOR OIL**

**DOSE—For adults, one tablespoonful. Children in proportion to age.**

**MATTHEWSON DRUG CO.**

**PRESCRIPTION DRUGGISTS**

**TWO ENTRANCES: 205 N. WASHINGTON AVENUE AND 103 W. AUSTIN STREET**

**PHONES: 741-742 REG. NO. 3288 MARSHALL, TEX.**

talked about old times, a man who reminded me of a Dallas Cowboy fullback sauntered in the front door, removed a boot and sock, and flopped a nasty foot on the checkout counter. He pointed a monstrous finger at a monstrous wart on his heel and said, "Wan-t'cha ta' remove that."

Slack-jawed, I just stood there and listened. Ken leaned in study, cut a quick glance to me, and winked. He then stepped around the counter and returned with a small dropper bottle, a pack of 3 × 4 gauze pads, and some tape. I watched as he placed a drop or two (of what he told me later was pure castor oil) on the wart, carefully covered the gruesome looking growth with the gauze, and strapped the whole thing down with tape. Ken then straightened his back and with authority running behind his words, said, "Leave that on and don't get it wet. Remove the bandage in two days, and bury it under your front porch. That'll be five dollars."

It amazed me the professional seriousness with which Ken approached the whole procedure. The man paid up, said, "Thanks," and hobbled out the door. He'd no sooner driven away than Ken broke into guffaws. "Come look at this," and he led me around the counter. Pasted on the wall above his desk were several prescriptions written by a local physician that read, "Remove wart, prn."

"I did this the first time as a prank on an old woman that owed me some money," Ken said. "When she went to the doctor a month later, those warts were gone, the skin was smooth, no scar, nothing. I couldn't believe it. Neither could Dr. Littlejohn."

Makes you wonder just how many pioneer medicines like castor oil were used to treat ailments that shouldn't have worked. Magic aside, in old Ken's and that Cajun medicine woman's defense, castor oil, like many pioneer meds, had a valid scientific basis for its action. The oils extracted from the castor bean contain triricinolein, which in the gut and on the skin break down in to its isomer, ricinoleic acid. Organic acids are keratolytic (break down keratin layers in skin). Furuncles (warts) are virus infections in keratin layers of the skin.

The usual dose in the good old days was two or thee beans,

chewed and chased with beer. The cathartic dose of expressed castor oil was, and still is, fifteen milliliters (one tablespoonful). The benefits of taking castor oil are well documented, but its disgusting taste has always been its major drawback. Everything from a few drops of sassafras oil or wintergreen or cinnamon has been tried, to no avail. Taken in orange juice with plenty of sugar added seems to have been the most tried and true method to get it down. Personally, I'd rather chew a couple of the beans and chase it with lots and lots of beer. Commercially, castor oil was used in the manufacture of the first decent soaps and later as a lubricant for the first internal combustion engines. (1; 4; 5; 6; 12–pp. 108–9)

## CHALK (1753 TO DATE)

Prepared chalk (calcium carbonate or carbonated lime) was used in frontier days in many forms. It was mixed with mercury to make "gray powder," which was used as a laxative, but in itself it was an efficient antacid. It was taken straight in powders and prepared in liquid forms with glycerin and honey and cinnamon water. Taken orally, chalk is relatively safe because very little (7 to 19 percent) is absorbed into the body; it remains in the intestinal tract. Large doses can build up and cause constipation. Adding camphor or menthol and applying it topically was used as a soothing drying agent on scalds and burns. Dry, it was used as a pharmaceutical necessity to granulate metals into malleable medicinal forms. Today, it is being touted as a convenient source of calcium. A rather mute point considering the percentages actually absorbed from the gut. Calcium carbonate, plain old chalk like your great grandmother used for acute indigestion (pyrosis) or your teacher used on the blackboard, is still the main ingredient in most chewable antacids like Tums and its inexpensive generic substitutes. The usual dose was five hundred to one thousand milligrams twice daily or as needed. (2–pp. 122, 193, 240, 87, 306; 60–p. 736).

## CHAMOMILE (1753 TO DATE)

Chamomile is derived from the flowering heads of the plants, *Matricaria chamomilla* and *Anthemis nobilis,* families Asteraceae and Compositae. Chamomile was used to treat digestive disorders, as a stomachic and an anti-inflammatory, for skin conditions, minor infections, pyrosis, and anxiety and restlessness. Extracts were used in inhalations, ointments, and lotions. It was popular in Germany as a ginseng-type remedy. The active ingredients were the flavonoids, apegenin and quercitin, bisabololoxides, matricin, hydroxycoumarines, and mucilages. Its main action may rest more on the combination of its constituents rather than a single agent. It was commonly prepared in tea form by boiling two to three teaspoonfuls in eight ounces of water, letting it steep, straining it, and taking it three or four times a day. The common dose of dry powder was one thousand milligrams three times daily; the fluid extract, one teaspoonful three times a day. (30–p. 83; 67–p. 83; 68–accessed September 29, 2002)

## CHARCOAL (1753 TO DATE)

Medicinal wood charcoal, official in the first pharmacopoeias, was preferentially prepared from willow and poplar trees. It was then powdered and standardized to increase its consistency and absorptive properties. Charcoal was also prepared by the destructive distillation of animal products. Due to availability and ease of production, official animal charcoal was replaced by wood charcoal. Also known as lamp black, cold black ash, and soot, charcoal has been used as a medicine for ages. Activated charcoal, the primary form used today, is still the choice as an antidote for orally ingested chemical toxins. Powdered charcoal has a large surface area, which absorbs and therefore prevents the gut from sopping up poisons. Technically, it interrupts the liver's recirculation of drugs in the gut and other compounds excreted into the bile. It was primarily used in conjunction with laxatives to help prevent bowel gas and lower belly discomforts. Soot mixed with sugar was applied topically as an antiseptic and styptic.

Another medicinal form of charcoal was coffee charcoal, a byproduct of the coffee industry. Roasting the outer portions of coffee beans into a char produced the final product. Medicinal coffee charcoal was used orally (in three-gram doses) for diarrhea and applied topically to treat festering wounds. Like soot, it was thought to have styptic properties, the effect of which was probably due more to the charcoals highly absorptive properties than its ability to stop bleeding, but who knows?

On vacation once to Colorado, my wife and I had the wonderful occasion to visit an old gold mining area. Beside a creek that ran slow with foul water stood a crudely constructed tower made of rock and wood. We were told that the old miner constructed this box back in the nineteenth century to filter the water to make it drinkable. He filled the inside of the contraption with charcoal chunks collected from his campfires and poured the bad water into the top. The good water that trickled through to a small holding area, he bottled and drank.

The biggest problem I see with medicinal charcoal was getting it down. If you've ever gotten chimney soot or lantern smut on your hands, you know how hard it is to remove. Finely powdered charcoal was often mixed with honey or syrup and taken. Imagine swallowing the stuff and the mess it had to have made on your teeth, tongue, and gums. The common oral dose of processed charcoal was one gram. (1–p. 140; 2–p. 98; 4–pp. 20, 306)

## CHAULMOOGRA OIL (1826–1955)

Chaulmoogra oil is a fixed oil expressed from the seeds of the plant *Hydrnocarpus anthelmintica*, family Flacourtiaceae. The oil of the chaulmoogra possesses a toxic affinity for *Mycobacterium leprae*, the bacterium that causes leprosy. For topical use, the oil was compounded into emulsions and ointments and also used for psoriasis, eczema, and skin disorders. Orally, it was taken to treat leprosy and as a sedative and an antipyretic. It was a notoriously nauseating emetic. In the later part of the nineteenth century, it was combined with resorcin and camphor and injected. The common dose was one milliliter. (1–p. 188)

## CHLORAL (1832 TO DATE)

Chloral, also known as chloral hydrate (1868 to date) and a Mickey Finn (1870 to date), was first synthesized in England in 1832. Chloral is a potent somnifacient (makes you sleep). Combining it with alcohol has a synergistic action (makes the drug even stronger). A dose of the drug was commonly five hundred milligrams. It took effect readily, within fifteen to thirty minutes, and lasted for seven to ten hours. Most syrups contained five hundred milligrams per five milliliters (teaspoonful). A standard medicine dropper was capable of delivering 2 to 2.5 milliliters; hence the name "knock-out drops" came into being. Two droppers full mixed in whiskey would knock out even the toughest of hombres. The drug has a slightly bitter taste that is easily covered with whiskey or fruit juice. In Chicago in the 1870s, a group of devious Irish tavern owners concocted what they called a Mickey Finn by mixing whiskey and chloral into a drink, which was used for the sole purpose of knocking a patron out so they could be robbed.

The name *chloral hydrate* came into being when the drug was marketed in the States in 1868 as the first therapeutically effective sleeping medicine. The drug's mode of action when taken internally was at first thought attributable to its being converted to chloroform in the body. This hypothesis didn't stand up to scrutiny. A metabolite known as urochloralic acid was later detected and studied by earlier investigators. Today, its action appears to be more related to a metabolite called trichloroethanol. Chloral's precise action on the central nervous system remains unclear to this day.

Chloral circulates in the blood and passes unchanged into breast milk. A nursing mother who took a dose could unknowingly and dangerously dose her child, too. (60–p. 1015)

## CHLOROFORM (1831 TO DATE)

Chloroform, trichloromethane, can be prepared in several ways: by reacting calcium hypochlorite with acetone, by the controlled chlorination of methane, and by the reduction of carbon tetrachloride with water and iron, the latter being the method used by frontier chemists. Pure chloroform decomposes on storage and should be prepared fairly fresh. Exposure to moisture and sunlight hastens its degradation. Adding alcohol greatly slows its decomposition.

A major advantage chloroform had over ether was that it wasn't flammable. At a time when most lighting was done with a candle and a coal oil lantern, this became a very important safety issue.

Exposed to heat and sunlight, many tonics and remedies went bad with time and took on a sour or rancid taste. Chloroform was an excellent solvent; added in tiny amounts to the old formulas, along with alcohol, it acted as a preservative to prevent vegetable constituents from "rotting" in the bottle. As an anesthetic, it was very potent, but it evaporated quickly. A cloth saturated with ounce or two and held over the nose acted within minutes. Anyone who has ever been put under by chloroform will tell you that it was a frightening experience, a smothering, panicky sensation, which made most people fight it before they went under. Once the patient was anesthetized, leaving the cloth over the nose and adding a few drops every minute or so kept them under.

It was made into a popular liniment by mixing powdered lye soap, camphor, oil of rosemary, alcohol, and water and used for everything from rash to rheumatism. Using chloroform as a topical medicinal agent was a rather mute effort since most of it evaporated within seconds. The camphor in the potions was the real therapeutic agent. However, the odor of chloroform could have had a psychological influence on the liniment's effectiveness. Anything that took your breath and left a hot sensation on the skin had to be strong enough to do some good.

Taken orally in tiny amounts, it had a carminative action. Adding menthol, anise, or camphor made it even better. It was prepared according to official compendiums in the form of chloroform water, dose one tablespoonful, and chloroform spirits, dose two milliliters. (2–pp. 58, 106, 204, 354)

## CHOKEBERRY

Chokeberry was the fruit of *Aronia medikus* and *Aronia melanocarpa*, family Rosaceae. Also known as black chokeberry or the chokeberry mountain ash, chokeberry has been used in folk medicine for centuries. The fruit was used as an anti-inflammatory, antirheumatic, diuretic, laxative, stomachic, and treatment for urinary complaints. The active ingredient, anthocyanin, has been proven to have significant antioxidant properties, which justifies its use in many of the old frontier tonics. (70–accessed October 2, 2002)

## CINNAMON (78 B.C. TO DATE)

Cinnamon is obtained from the bark, leaves, and stem tips of *Laurus cinnamomum*, *Zeylanicum cinnamomum*, *Cassia cinnamomum*, and *Burmanni cinnamomum*, family Lauraceae. The plant parts are gathered from young trees (usually less than six years old), dried, and then ground into a fine powder. Internally, it was used as a carminative in a dose of 0.25 gram. Cinnamon oil (1820 to date) was steam distilled from the leaves and twigs of *C. cassia.* As a medicinal, it was used as a carminative, antiseptic, antiflatulant, antistimulant, and antidiarrheal. The oil was dosed at 0.1 milliliter.

Cinnamaldehyde, the active ingredient, increases blood flow and has antipyretic, antibacterial, and antifungal activity. Cinnamon bark is a urinary irritant that, technically, is thought to work in premature ejaculation by increasing the penile vibratory threshold and reducing the amplitude of penile somatosensory potentials (the ability to consciously delay ejaculation). "Penile vibratory threshold." I didn't know I had one of them. My "somatosensory potentials" sure seem depleted these days, too.

Cinnamon was prepared in a spirit by adding one part of cinnamon oil to ten parts of alcohol and dosed at one milliliter; prepared into a water by adding two milliliters of the oil to a liter of water. The usual oral dose of the water was fifteen milliliters (one tablespoonful). Nowhere, anywhere, could I find a dose for increasing penile vibratory thresholds and somatosensory potentials—sorry. (1–pp. 214–19; 2–pp. 58, 111, 256, 352; 4–p. 286)

## CLOVE OIL (1753 TO DATE)

Also known as oleum caryophylli, clove oil is the volatile oil that is steam distilled from the dried flower buds of the tree, *Eugenia caryophyllus*, family Myrtaceae. Clove oil was used as a dental obtundant (having the ability to dull tooth pain). Orally it was taken as a carminative, as an antiemetic (stops vomiting), for diarrhea and halitosis (bad breath), and as a stomachic. Topically it was applied as an anesthetic for "dry sockets" in dentistry. Eugenol, one of the active ingredients of clove oil, was and is still used for dental pain. Clove oil was used to flavor toothpicks. The ingredient, eugenyl acetate in it, has antihistamine and antispasmodic properties and inhibits both gram-negative and gram-positive bacteria. It was used in mouthwashes (containing 1 to 5 percent of the oil), prepared in a fluidextract (dosed at five to thirty drops orally), and as the pure oil (dosed orally at one to five drops). Clove bark (*Cassia caryophyllatta*) was used in tonics and stomachic formulas as a flavoring and carminative. (1–pp. 219, 231; 4–p. 294)

## COAL OIL (KEROSENE) (1753 TO DATE)

Also known as petrolatum bitumen and kerosene, coal oil is a volatile oil distilled from petroleum and other hydrocarbons. Aside from its role as an illuminant, coal oil was used as a soak for puncture wounds, as a base for liniments, and as a rubefacient. Kerosene, as it later came to be called, was a pioneer's primary antiseptic. Much like turpentine, it was used to treat injuries inflicted by rusty objects (to prevent lockjaw). A block of camphor dissolved in a lard bucket of coal oil made a fine veterinary liniment. It was used as a base for many wart remedies and practically everything else on the farm. You got a cut, you dabbed it with coal oil; you or your farm animal stepped on a nail or got snake bit, you soaked it in coal oil; bott flies pestering your horses, you wiped their backs with coal oil; your lamp went out, you filled it with coal oil; you needed to burn a pile of brush, you doused it with coal oil; your wife got mad at you, you patted her lightly . . . and apologized.

## COCA-COLA (1886 TO DATE)

Coke, as we know it, was discovered by a pharmacist/doctor named John Stith Pemberton in 1886. His cola leaf drink, also referred to as his wine cola, was an imitation of a coca–wine drink originally developed in 1883 by a Frenchman named Angelo Mariania. Pemberton's formula, however, proved to be superior as a medicine to stop and prevent nausea. The unhealthy pharmacist was also a morphine addict. His use of the thick, black syrup for nausea may have been one of his reasons for developing Coke as a medicine. In 1887, Pemberton sold part ownership in the product to several investors, none of which had the time to market, make, or sell it, so they in turn got out. One co-owner, Willis Venable, gave his portion to Joseph Jacobs, a pharmacist. Pemberton in the meantime found three more investors and moved the company to Atlanta, Georgia, where they produced Pemberton's wonderful medicine. After Pembertons's death, Asa Chandler acquired sole ownership and in turn became the richest man in Atlanta selling what became the most popular soft drink in America. The popular modern product Emetrol (used for nausea) is based on the same therapeutic premise as original Coke syrup.

## COCOA BUTTER (1863 TO DATE)

Cocoa butter, also known as theobroma oil, is the fat obtained from the seeds (cocoa beans) of *Theobroma cacoa*, family Sterculiaceae. Cocoa butter was a yellowish white solid fat that had a bland taste and a chocolate odor. It was used primarily as a base for suppositories because it was relatively innocuous and melted at slightly above room temperature. It was applied topically as an emollient and softening agent for dry skin. The only time it was taken orally was when someone misunderstood the directions on the proper use of a suppository and chewed it up. In those instances, it reportedly had a "yucky" taste.

Cocoa, from cocoa beans, the food of the gods (better known as chocolate), was used medicinally as a stimulant (it contains small amounts of caffeine); as an expectorant for lung congestion; for liver, bladder, and kidney ailments; and as a general tonic added to syrups. The active ingredients were tannins, theobromine, caffeine, and tyramine. (1–p. 192; 4–298)

## COD LIVER OIL (1851 TO DATE)

Cod liver oil, also known as oleum morrhuae, is a fixed oil obtained from the fresh livers of the cod fish, *Gadus morrhua*, family Gadidae, a fish that inhabits the north Atlantic Ocean and spawns in late winter and spring in New England. Early pioneers harvested the fish, cleaned and salted the meat, then threw the livers, gallbladders and all, into huge vats to "rot." The crude oil that rose to the top of the containers was skimmed off, strained, and packaged for use as medicine. The main medicinal constituents were vitamin

A and vitamin D. The oil's primary use was for rickets, a disease marked by bending and distortion of the bones under muscular action—a condition most characterized in frontier times as "old man bowleggedness," which was a misnomer that actually affected young and old alike who were deficient in vitamins A and D. The oil was applied topically for eczema and psoriasis, heat rash, gauld, and diaper rash. It was combined with zinc oxide in ointments. White's Cod Liver Oil Concentrate and White's A&D Ointment are still available today. (1–p. 400; 10–p. 18)

## COLUMBA (1753 TO DATE)

Also known as calumba, Texas sarsaparilla, and yellor parilla, columba was the dried root of *Columba palmata* and *Minispermum canadense*, family Minespermaceae. Columba root has a persistent bitter, almost acrid taste. The medicine was used in many folk remedies as a bitter, which had gastrotonic and stomachic activity. The active ingredients in columba were the alkaloids, alumbin, chasmanthin, columbamine, berberine, and minespermum. Texas sarsaparilla had tonic, diuretic, laxative, alterative, and nervine properties. Externally it was decocted and as an embrocation applied to treat the swelling from gouty, arthritic inflammations.

The powdered root of both *M. canadense* and *C. palmata* was given straight in 0.5-dram doses, in fluid extracts, in 0.5-dram doses, and in decoctions, one to four ounces three times daily. Because of their morphinelike side effects, they seldom see use today as medicines. (6–p. 1128; 71–accessed October 4, 2002; 72–accessed October 4, 2002)

## COPPER (2600 B.C. TO DATE)

Elemental copper is a mineral known to be necessary to human metabolism. As early as 2600 B.C., copper was listed in the *Papyrus*, an Egyptian medical reference, as an element that the body requires but cannot produce on its own. Just as early physicians were able to derive medicinals from plants, they relied on metals like copper, manganese, and zinc for their healing properties. Copper was, in ancient times, found useful for its antifungal and antibacterial powers. The green pigment spoken of in those earliest of pharmacopoeias was likely malachite, a native carbonate of copper found in copper ores.

The metal's first role in helping strengthen the immune system was published in 1867 when it was reported that workers in copper mines, during cholera epidemics, were immune to the disease. Such evidence led early researchers to strongly believe that copper and its compounds could not only cure disease but also help prevent it. Copper acetate prepared into a salve with hog lard was used to treat and prevent arthritis. Wearing copper jewelry was thought to help strengthen the body's immunity to rheumatism and cancer. Copper arsenate was used for chronic diarrhea, dysentery, and cholera. Black copper oxide was mixed with honey and taken to purge the system of pinworms. Dilute solutions were used as drops in the nose for congestion, in the eyes for grittiness and burning, as a mouthwash and gargle for ulcerations in the mouth, and for sore throat.

The belief is that redistributing copper in the body plays a significant role in the body's response mechanisms to disease, a medical capacity that is essential to the healing process. This elevation of copper in diseased states is suspected to account for a natural synthesis of copper-dependent proteins and enzymes that regulate biochemical responses to tissue trauma and stress. Copper sulfate (460 B.C. to date), also known as blue vitriol and blue copperas, was mentioned in the early medical texts as a sprinkle treatment for flesh wounds. An effective management of venereal disease was prepared by cooking pepper, myrrh, and saffron with copper oxide, first by pounding the copper compound in wine and heating it until dry. The powder was then taken orally. For ulcers and bedsores, copper sulfate was moistened to a soft consistency with rose oil and applied topically.

One of the nation's most prominent cowboys, the old Duke himself, John Wayne, wore a copper bracelet to help strengthen his immune system. Unfortunately, it didn't cure him, the cancer finally won, but who knows how long that bracelet prolonged his life?

Today, more than 140 copper complexes of compounds like ibuprofen and aspirin, when tested on animals, have been shown to be more active than their parent compounds. Studies are also showing a relationship between copper levels and heart disease. Researchers have found, too, that copper retards cancer in mice. Lately, copper complexes have been shown to heal gastric ulcers and wounds sooner. Anticonvulsant activity of other medications is enhanced by copper's presence.

The human brain contains more copper than any other organ of the body, except the liver, where it is stored, but unfortunately there is no proof that supplementing copper is beneficial for people who eat a healthy, normal diet. It does seem odd, though, that as long ago as 2600 B.C., they already knew some of what we're finding out today about many old remedies like copper. Who knows what tomorrow's research will show? (4–p. 323; 60–p. 748; 73–accessed October 7, 2002)

## CORN SILK (1700 TO DATE)

Corn silk contains tannins known to have astringent effects and cryptoxanthins, which have vitamin-based, alterative effects on the body. Typical recorded doses were about a teaspoonful of the crushed and crumbled or powdered silks three times daily, or one cup of tea prepared much the same way as Grandma did, taken several times daily for prostatitis, cystitis, urethritis, and nocturnal enuresis (old man's dribble.)

Corn silk as a drug was the dried threads from around the ear, prepared from *Zea mays*, family Gramineae. Orally, it was used to treat acute and chronic inflammation of the urinary tract. The Chinese used it as a diuretic and to treat a bad heart.

## COTTON

The applicable part of the cotton plant was the bark of the roots of *Gossypium herbaceum*, family Malvaceae. It was dried and pulverized and then taken to stimulate menstrual flow and—get this—as a male contraceptive. The active part of the plant was gossypo, which was later found to be more readily available from the cotton's seeds than from the bark. Gossypol's male contraceptive action was due to its inhibition of an enzyme called lactate dehydrogenase X, which is essential to the liveliness of sperm metabolism. Gossypol may also have inhibited prostaglandin synthesis. The major drawback was that in many instances it worked too well and caused irreversible sterility. The oral dose for male contraception was twenty milligrams daily for three months, followed by a weekly maintenance dose of fifty to one hundred milligrams. You didn't know just how soft and cool cotton really was, now did you? (4–pp. 507–8)

## COW'S MILK COLOSTRUM

Also known as bovine colostrum, cow's milk colostrums were used orally to stimulate the growth and health of sickly children. High in protein, carbohydrates, fat, vitamins, and immunity factors, the "first milk" did indeed make a puny kid perkier. One cup four times a day was the usual dose.

Because of colostrum's enhanced immunity qualities, it is used today for enhanced athletic training. Studies are also under way to determine its possible use in AIDS-related *Chlostridium parvum* diarrhea. (4–pp. 174–75)

## CREAM OF TARTAR (1753 TO DATE)

Cream of tartar, potassium bitartrate, was prepared by processing the crude residues deposited in the bottoms of wine casks during fermentation of grapes. The dregs contained about 80 percent

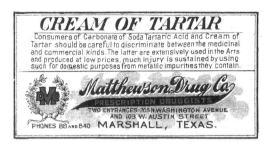


potassium bitartrate. It was largely used in baking powders. With sulfur added, it made the popular laxative Sulfur and Cream of Tartar Tablets. It was also used in the production of hard candy. The usual dose was two grams. (60–p. 745)

## CREOSOTE (1842 TO DATE)

Creosote was a mixture obtained from wood tar by the destructive distillation of beechwood and other trees. Upon distillation, the heavy layer of tar was treated with sodium carbonate, potassium hydroxide, and sulfuric acid and collected into containers. The final product was yellowish oil with a smoky odor and caustic taste. Its primary use was as a disinfectant and in topical treatments for psoriasis and skin irritations. Orally, in 0.25-milliliter doses, it was used as an expectorant.

Wagon wheels were lubricated with various tars and petroleum products obtained from open pits containing crude oils and tars. Continuous abrasion and heat exerted on these crude lubricants produced a rude form of creosote. An ointment prepared from this "burned" axle grease and powdered sulfur was used by pioneers as a rough-and-ready topical antibiotic.

## CROTON OIL (1753–1947)

Croton oil was obtained from the seeds of the Euphorbiaceae family of plants. The word *croton* means "bug" in Greek because of the seed's dark brown color and shape. The seeds originally came from a tree indigenous to Asia. Later, the trees were commercially cultivated in the East Indies and shipped to the States. Once expressed from the seed, the fixed oil was a yellowish, almost fluorescent liquid that had a faint acidic odor. Croton oil was so irritating when applied to skin that it caused puss-filled blisters resembling pimples. There was only one cathartic more powerful than croton oil, and that was colocynth, which saw little use as a medicine.

Nowhere in my research was I able to verify an age-old story about croton oil that tells of a farmer who got tired of thieves stealing his watermelons, so he placed a sign on his fence that read, "One of these melons has croton oil in it." The fable goes that the next morning he returned to find someone had marked through the "one" on his sign and wrote, "Two."

Fiction, fact, or joke, the old story stresses how strong croton oil was known to be. Used when other cathartics failed, the usual oral dose of croton oil was one to two drops (0.06 milliliter) placed in liquid, on sugar or bread and taken at bedtime. Puts a whole new light on the old saying "Rise and shine," don't it? (2; 4; 5; 6)

## DANDELION (1753 TO DATE)

The whole plant, roots, puff, stems leaves, and all of *Taraxacum officinale*, family Asteraceae, were used as medicine in both pioneer and frontier times. Orally, it was used to stimulate bile flow, for indigestion, for constipation, for flatulence, and as a tonic. Asian frontiersmen used it to treat cancer, for rheumatic inflammations, gout, and stiff joints. Dried and roasted, dandelion was used as a "poor boy's" coffee. Dandelion contains taraxacin, a bitter component, which is responsible for increasing bile flow. In teas, the concoction acted as a diuretic, and as a stomachic. The aboveground parts of the dandelion plant contain more vitamin A than carrots. The typical dose of the leaf was four to ten grams. A tea was prepared by boiling four to ten grams (approximately one to two teaspoonfuls) in four ounces of water. It was steeped for ten minutes, then strained and consumed. A liquid extract prepared by mixing equal weights of alcohol and ground dried roots was dosed at two to eight milliliters. It is still an active ingredient in Lydia Pinkham's famous vegetable potion. (4–p. 360)

## DEER

The Native American influence on frontier medicine was as profound as that of the Europeans. But the Asians, though merely hinted at here and there in historical passages, had a significant effect on frontier medicine and survival. The typical role of the Chinese frontiersman was that of "wash lady or "wash man"—the ones who did the laundry. They were a clean society and did that job well. However, on the medicine end, they had more influence than many people realize.

The Chinese frontiersman's basic medical philosophy was that of yin and yang, which professes that cosmic forces control life's processes and all natural phenomena. Their theory was that illness was an imbalance between this yin and yang. Along with the turtle and the crane, the deer was recognized as a symbol of luck. Perhaps the most important animal to the Chinese frontiersman's medicine chest was the deer, which to them was a mark of longevity. The most valued portion was the fleshy velvet that grew on the deer's horns, deer velvet (168 B.C. to date). This soft covering that nourished the stag's growing antler grew rapidly. Its capacity to regenerate was what made the covering so unique. An important Chinese volume from 1596 written by Li Shi Zhen titled *Grand Materio Medico* lists deer velvet to tonify yang by increasing its vital forces and to treat arthritis. Dried and powdered deer velvet was used to cure exhaustion, increase the body's resistance to infection, and improve physical strength. Studies show that consuming deer velvet improves memory, stamina, aids osteoporosis, and helps a person recover from physical trauma.

Deer velvet contains a variety of ingredients: sulfur, sodium, phosphorus, iron, magnesium, phospholipids, and gylcolipids, but the most significant effectual appears to be the organic combinations of growth factors that stimulate fleshy regeneration. It being natural and primarily flesh, there was a wide safety margin in taking it. It was removed from the antler, cured, dried and powdered, sometimes soaked in wine, or prepared in a tincture. In some instances the entire horn was removed, ground up, and prepared as a medicine.

As a general tonic, the dose of the pure cured velvet was five hundred milligrams daily; for rheumatism and arthritis, up to one gram daily.

Deer velvet is undergoing significant study today in other countries and is being made available abroad in encapsulated forms to treat arthritis, strengthen the immune system, and as a natural way to improve the stamina of athletes. I'm told it is also touted to promote youthfulness and to treat impotence in both men and women. Oh, deer.

The use of deer musk as a medicine goes back five thousand years. Japanese Samurai carried musk pouches to protect them from evil during battle. The oily, odiferous exudates from the male deer's glands that grew on the insides of its back leg were used by pioneer Asians to treat stroke, convulsions, heart pain, as a relaxant, and to treat ulcerations. The word *musk* is derived from the ancient Indian word *muskah* which means "testicles."

Most frontier musk was harvested after killing a deer by removing the gland, soaking it in whiskey overnight, and then squeezing out the oily residue. Asian frontiersmen and women used musk to stimulate the "life force" in the body and as a catalyst for other medicines. It was also used to make perfumes, which were supposed to have aphrodisiac properties. This makes sense since the gland's secretions did indeed contain natural pheromones. (4–p. 363; 74–accessed October 14, 2002)

## DEER BALLS

Also known as puff balls, Hart's truffle, or smut balls, deer balls were the aerial parts and spores of *Lycoperdon* spp., family Gasteromycetes. Orally and topically, the spores were the active part of the mushroom. Deer ball spores, or "smut," contains amino acids, sterol, glucosamine, enzymes, and urea. My other brother Don and I used to enjoy drop-kicking them and watching them smoke. Grandma Leorah told us never to breathe that smoke "'cause it would make us sick." I looked that up. She was right. The inhaled spores were notorious for clinging to the lung linings and causing a form of pneumonia. And back in frontier times, any form of pneumonia was capable of being fatal.

Prepared in an alcoholic extract, the medicine was taken for nosebleed and applied for skin disorders. A common frontier method of preparation was to remove or pick the whole mushroom, keeping its hull intact, poke a small hole in it, and pour it full of whiskey. It was then swirled, left to set a minute, and poured into a dropper bottle. (4–p. 866)

## DIGITALIS (1753 TO DATE)

Also known as foxglove and dead man's bells, digitalis was the dried leaf of *Digitalis purpurea*, family Scrophulariaceae. The plant was a biennial herb whose internal use didn't really come into vogue as a well-known and well-used heart medicine until 1776. Foxglove contained several glycosides, one of which was digitoxin, the most medically significant heart drug of all times. Powdered, the plant was used to increase the tone of cardiac muscle (it made the heart beat stronger). The most significant attribute of digitalis was that the therapeutic range between effectiveness and death was very narrow. Because of the drug's stimulant action on the heart by improving circulation, which it does in the kidney, too, it was included in many earlier remedies as a diuretic. A major problem with the digitalis plant was that once dried, it often was confused with other herbs and was a dangerous and deadly adulterant. Powdered, the dose of whole leaf foxglove was 1.5 grams divided over twenty-four to forty-eight hours. Maintenance dose was one hundred milligrams daily. It was often prepared in an alcoholic tincture that was dosed from two to twenty drops daily.

Historically, digitalis wasn't used so much for the heart as it was as a diuretic for swelling feet and legs, as an emetic, and to treat epileptic seizures, tuberculosis, and constipation. It was also applied topically to burns. A tonic containing foxglove was indeed a deadly elixir, particularly during a period of time when people thought that if a little did good, a lot would do better. Unfortunately, for the elderly or the infant, better, likely as not, meant going to heaven. (1–pp. 94–103; 4–372)

## DIRT

Cowboys have always been close to the earth. The land grinds its way into a cowboy's body. Wind blown dust comes in through his eyes and nose. Mud and gravel gets between his toes. True grit winds its way into his biscuits, into his tobacco, and into his character. But on occasion, he rubs it on or swallows it on purpose.

Dirt in the form of calamine, pascalite, dolomite, kaolin, and Dover's clays were and still are forms of medicine. Topically, clay was mixed into poultices and used as osmotic emollients, as drying agents in dusting powders, and taken internally for dysentery and diarrhea.

The purest form of medicinal clay came from the Cliffs of Dover in Europe (don't confuse Dover's clay with Dover's powder, which contained opium and ipecac and was used as a diaphoretic). Pure consistencies of white, gray, or red clays obtained here in the states were also used in folk medicines.

Clay is nature's purest form of dirt. Formed thirty million years ago, over the centuries, calcium from limestone formations combined with other minerals—aluminum, manganese, cobalt, copper, magnesium, and silica—and slowly, through oxidation, were converted to an even consistency. Further enriched by abundant plant life (decomposed tissues, bones, hides, and hair of many prehistoric animals) added proteins and amino acids to the pasty formations.

Bentonite (calcium bentonite), also known as pascalite or white Indian clay, was used as medicine long before the coming of the white man. Native Crow, Arapahoe, Blackfoot, Shoshone, and Sioux Indians taught the white man the healing powers of clay. The Indians called white clay *ee-wah-kee*, which meant "the mud that heals." There is a story about a white man who accompanied a Shoshone chief on a buffalo hunt in 1888 and fell horribly ill. The Shoshone medicine man rubbed the sick man with herbs and made him drink white clay dissolved in water. The man totally recovered from his illness.

The name *pascalite* comes from a French-Canadian trapper named Emile Pascal who was the first white man to mine and promote clay as a medicine. He sold the "pure dirt" as a treatment for raw and chapped skin, gaulds, rashes, insect bites, and stomach troubles. Mud was heated, mixed with herbs (e.g., prairie sage), and applied for bruised and sore muscles. Mixed into ointments it was applied to hemorrhoids. Clay was used as an abrading agent not only to cleanse and scrub pots and pans but to remove "proud and stinky dead-flesh" that formed on a man who had gone for months without a bath. The awareness developed by exposing fresh and sensitive skin was invigorating and just plain made a man feel "good all over." Our modern-day Lava soap with its pumice is a hand-me-down of the warm clay baths pioneers used to take.

When taken orally, as it absorbed water, clay expanded many times its dry weight. A tablespoonful of pure clay, combined with a tablespoon of ground flaxseeds in water, made an excellent topical drying agent for oozing sores like poison ivy. Calamine, too, was nothing more than a type of clay.

Kaolin (hydrated aluminum silicate), also called porcelain clay, has been used orally for centuries. Refined by washing crude kaolin clay with acids and water, with the coarser particles separated into a fine powder and combined with pectin-forming agents and/or paregoric or tincture of opium, the thick suspension made an excellent oral product to treat diarrhea and stomach cramps. Kaolin is still used today as the FDA-approved product, known to many if not to all as Kaopectate.

Dolomite (dolomitic limestone) is also a refined dirt that is still used as natural elemental mineral sources of both calcium and magnesium. (4–p. 378; 4–p. 623; 75–accessed October 14, 2002)

## DOGWOOD (1820 TO DATE)

American dogwood, often called boxwood or rose willow, is a tree, *Cornus florida*, family Cornaceae. The dogwood tree has always held folklore favor and a mystique of marvel:

**The Legend of the Dogwood**

*The beautiful Dogwood once was as mighty as the oak.*
*The Romans used it for a cross on which to stake the savior's son.*
*Having heard this, God seized the tree in anger.*
*Because of the tree's sorrow over the cruel duty it performed,*
*With compassion, God opted to spare the dogwood an eternity of doom.*
*Henceforth, he ordained that the tree shall grow slender and twisted so that the wood could never again be used as a cross.*
*"For penitence," he bequeathed, "ye shall bear blossoms in the shape of a cross. On that cross shall appear a crown of thorns and nail prints stained with red so the world can see that it was you who carried my son to Calvary."*

The bark of the dogwood used in pioneer medicines contains alcohol soluble glycosides similar to quinine. Indians used the bark and roots for malaria and extracted a red dye from its roots. It was used in tonics and fluid extracts for headaches and fever, for fatigue, and as an appetite stimulant. In high doses, it was capable of suppressing a rapid heartbeat. By 1936, dogwood had fallen from all official listings as an accepted medicinal. It still is, however, an ingredient in Lydia E. Pinkham's famous herbal compound, which is, or was, available from drugstores at the time of this book's printing. (1–p. 166; 4–p. 50; 11–p. 14)

## EPHEDRINE (MA HUANG) (1898 TO DATE)

*Ephedra sinica* and *E. equisetina*, family Gnetaceae, also known as ephedra or ma huang, as a medicine was the aboveground parts of the plant. Ephedra has been used in China for over five thousand years. The plant is a low (usually less than three feet tall) bush that is nearly leafless. The best part was the young dried branches. There are two medically significant principal alkaloids in ephedra—ephedrine and pseudoephedrine, both of which directly simulate the nervous system, increasing blood pressure, heart rate, and constricting the blood vessels. Ephedra has diuretic and uterine-contracting properties. Asian immigrants introduced it to the West as a stimulant and diuretic and to treat colds, fever, chills, and headaches. Synthetically derived pseudoephedrine is available today as the product Sudafed. (1–p. 367; 4–p. 400; 10–p. 184c)

## EPSOM SALT (1753 TO DATE)

Magnesium sulfate was obtained from natural sources. It was abundant in the form of double salts with alkali metals in mines. It was highly effective as a saline laxative. The salt is not absorbed in-

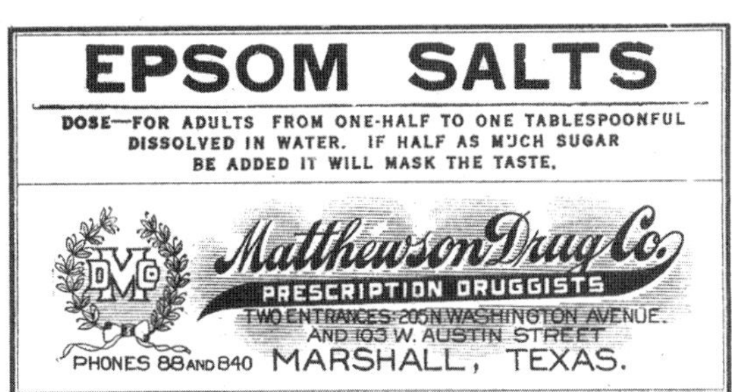
EPSOM SALTS
DOSE—FOR ADULTS FROM ONE-HALF TO ONE TABLESPOONFUL DISSOLVED IN WATER. IF HALF AS MUCH SUGAR BE ADDED IT WILL MASK THE TASTE.
MDC
Matthewson Drug Co.
PRESCRIPTION DRUGGISTS
TWO ENTRANCES 205 N. WASHINGTON AVENUE.
AND 103 W. AUSTIN STREET
PHONES 88 AND 840 MARSHALL, TEXAS.

ternally from the intestinal tract and thus draws water into the gut. By the sheer increase in fluid bulk, it promotes the motor activity of the bowel. It is nauseous to taste; drinking it cold or in orange juice helped get it down. Diluted in water and applied cold, by submersion of an extremity or saturated on cloth compresses, it served as a poultice for inflamed, arthritic-type ailments. Applied hot (one pound to a pint of hot water and soaked or on a compress), it was used to treat deep-seated, puncture-style skin infections. Usual oral dose was fifteen grams.

Glauber's salt, sodium sulfate (1753 to date), also often referred to as pioneer Epsom salt, occurred naturally in various minerals, in salt brines, and in various mineral springs. It, too, was a saline laxative and a topical anti-inflammatory. The usual oral dose was fifteen grams. (60–pp. 745–46)

## ERGOT (1820–1947)

*Claviceps purpurea*, family Hypocreaceae, better known as ergot, was the dried, hard, thick-walled, blackish mass formed by fungi on rye plants. This fungus periodically invaded rye fields, contaminating it. Inasmuch as ergot was such a potent constrictor of blood vessels, it having been a contaminant in bread was responsible for severe gangrene outbreaks in earlier times. Commonly referred to as St. Anthony's fire, the disease became epidemic in the 1600s. As a medicine, it didn't really become popular until early in the twentieth century. Ergot stimulates uterine contractions and possesses potent blood vessel constrictive properties. The black smut from rye grass, applied to wounds, stopped bleeding quite effectively. Ergot and its derivatives are used in modern migraine prescription remedies. (1–p. 353; 4–p. 404)

## ETHER (1275 TO DATE)

A product called sweet vitriol was discovered by a Spanish chemist named Raymundus Lullius in 1275. In 1730, a German scientist, W. G. Frobenius renamed it ether. Before its anesthetic properties were fully understood, sweet vitriol was used to treat catarrhal fever, bladder calculus (bladder stones), scurvy, and lung inflammations. A doctor named Crawford Williamson Long who hailed from Jefferson, Georgia, on March 30, 1842, first used ether as a surgical anesthetic to remove tumors from the neck of a patient. But since Dr. Long didn't publish his results in accepted journals, credit for ether's first use officially went to W. T. G. Morton, another physician. The first hospital operation using ether was performed in 1846, in Boston, at the College of Massachusetts.

Ether was an additive in many pioneer and frontier remedies but lost favor to the less flammable chloroform. Ether was an ingredient (as an expectorant/carminative) in the popular Chamberlain's Colic Remedy for flatulence and wind colic. Wind colic was defined in an old medical dictionary as "pain in the bowels due to their distension with air or gas." After having raised three boys (four if you include me), my wife would loved to have had access to that old remedy. (12–p. 108; 77–accessed October 18, 2002)

## EUCALYPTUS (1852 TO DATE)

Eucalyptus, *Eucalyptus globulus*, family Mytaceae, is a volatile oil that is steam distilled from the fresh leaves of the tree. The use of eucalyptus came to the Americas from Australia in 1852, primarily from enslaved aborigines. The aborigines had used the plant and its oil to aid in healing wounds and for fever. It was inhaled to treat asthma, whooping cough, bronchitis, and emphysema. It was a fragrant additive in remedies used to treat colds, aches, and pains. Infusions from the plant's leaves had bacterial and decongestant activity. It was also used as an insect repellant. The active ingredient, eucalyptol, stimulates the production of saliva and activates the swallowing reflex.

A typical dose of the powered leaf was a cup of tea prepared by steeping a teaspoonful in a cup of boiling water and straining. A 1:1 fluidextract using whiskey was dosed at a teaspoonful four times a day as a stimulant, as a mouthwash to relieve bleeding gums, and for rheumatism. The steam from the concoction was breathed for colds and asthma. Today, the primary use of eucalyptus is as a flavoring and as a scent in aromatherapy. (1–p. 245; 4–p. 407; 60–p. 1233)

## FENNEL (1820–1960)

Fennel is the dried ripe fruit of *Foeniculum vulgare*, family Umbelliferae. The plant was a perennial herb indigenous to Europe, Asia, India, and Japan. The powdered fruit was taken orally to enhance lactation, facilitate birth, promote menstruation, increase libido, and as an aromatic stimulant and stomachic. It was added to colic remedies for children. Prepared in a poultice, it was used to treat snakebites and as a flavoring agent. The fruits are a rich source of vitamin C, beta-carotene, magnesium, calcium, and iron. Anethole, the active ingredient, relieves bronchial secretions, promotes gastrointestinal motility, and in high doses acts as an antispasmodic. The typical medicinal dose of fennel, orally, was a heaping teaspoonful per day or as a tea, one cup three times daily, which was prepared by steeping a teaspoonful of powdered fennel for ten minutes in eight ounces of boiling water, straining, and taking. A tincture prepared with equal parts of powder and whiskey was dosed at a teaspoonful per day. Oil expressed from the seeds was often mixed with honey and used as a carminative, stomachic, and for upper respiratory congestion in children. Fennel was often added to sausage to give it that "Italian" taste. (1–p. 239; 4–p. 424)

## FIGS (1820–1936)

Also known as ficus, figs as a medicine were the partially dried fruit of the fig tree, *Ficus carica*, family Moraceae. Crude fig was used as a laxative and demulcent. Figs contain large amounts of sugar, which when incorporated into laxative potions made the products pleasant tasting and easy to take, particularly for children. Most patent remedies containing fig also contained small amounts alcohol to prevent "souring" of the product. Figs undergo a natural fermentive process to form ficin (spelled f-*i*-c-i-n) a fermentive, proteolytic enzyme (an organic agent that digests protein). Applied to fresh meat, ficin was the first tenderizer used by the meat industry. Prepared ficin was such a potent digestive enzyme that it couldn't be used topically; it irritated and burned too bad. Instead, it was taken orally as an ascaricide (killed roundworms) and in trichuriasis (killed whipworms). The ficin enzyme literally dissolved the worms inside the gut and caused purging, which helped expel them. (I've always wanted to write that—"a ficin enzyme." Sorry.) (1–pp. 63, 422; 4–p. 433)

## FLAXSEED (2300 B.C. TO DATE)

Also known as linseed, flaxseed was the dried ripe seeds of *Linum usitatissimum*, family Linaceae. With the possible exception of cotton, flax fibers were of great economic value when made into cloth. Fabric made from the fibers of flax plants dates back to Egyptian tomb times. The cloth that covered mummies was made from flax fibers. Whole flaxseeds were often encased in many tombs.

The most memorable or significant use of flaxseeds as a pioneer medicine was to aid in the removal of foreign objects from the eye. The outer hull contains mucilage, which swells when it comes in contact with water. Moistened first in warm water, the seed immediately became slick, like a watermelon seed. Placed in the eye on the outer orbit as it slid around when the eye was blinked, it picked up grit and foreign objects like a magnet. Working it to the corner near the nose and sliding it out, the seed and the trash adhering to it were easily removed.

Flaxseed oil, also known as linseed oil, taken internally was a laxative, protective, and demulcent. For use in paint, linseed oil was boiled with metal salts, which hastened its drying time and made it an excellent paint and varnish base. Boiling the oil, however, made it toxic. Only the "raw, unboiled linseed oil" could be used medicinally.

The usual dose of linseed (flaxseed) was a tablespoonful of the whole or bruised seeds (not ground) with six ounces of water taken two to three times daily, followed by ample fluid intake. Topically, a finely powdered form with added herbs (camphor, sage or such) was used in hot poultices and soothing compresses. (1–p. 182; 4–p. 440)

## GARLIC (1820–1936)

Yes, plain old garlic, the one that gives you bad breath, was recognized in official compendiums (U.S.P. 1820–1863 and N.F. 1916–1936) as a carminative and expectorant. The raw cloves of *Allium sativum*, family Alliaceae, hold about 0.25 percent of a volatile oil, which contains a sulfur compound called alliin. Other active ingredients include allylpropyl disulfide, cysteines, mercaptocysteines, and s-allylcysteine. A vaginal product of garlic mixed with yogurt was used for vaginitis. These ingredients in garlic have been shown in modern analysis to have antibacterial, diaphoretic, expectorant, antispasmodic, and blood clot–reducing properties. The stinky herb was used for centuries to treat colds, fever, coughs, snakebites, and even as (provided both parties partook of it) an aphrodisiac. Garlic is undergoing intense study today for its ability to help prevent coronary heart disease. (1–p. 250; 4–p. 465)

## GENTIAN ROOT (1820 TO DATE)

The dried root (rhizome) of *Gentiana lutea*, family Gentianaceae, also known as American gentian and buckbean, was classified as a bitter that was used in tonic remedies for digestive disorders. Gentian root contains three bitter glycosides, gentopiricin, gentiamarin, and gentisin or gentianic acid, which are responsible for their digestive juice stimulation and anti-inflammatory activity. The usual dose was formerly listed as one gram of the powdered root three times daily. A tea prepared by steeping a heaping teaspoonful of the powder in twelve ounces of water and strained was taken three times a day. The usual dose of a fluidextract was a teaspoonful daily. Asian frontiersmen used gentian root for jaundice, headache, and rheumatoid arthritis. (1–p. 155; 4–p. 469)

## GENTIAN VIOLET (1856 TO DATE)

Also known as basic violet and aniline purple, gentian violet was a purple dye prepared from coal tar. The active ingredient in crude gentian violet was aniline. Gentian violet killed bacteria. In earlier times it was applied topically to burns and to infected lesions. Taken orally, it killed pinworms and relieved urinary irritations. Gentian violet was incorporated in vaginal douches and vaginal inserts for *Monilia* infections. As a vermifuge, it was dosed at fifty milligrams three times daily. In 1 percent solutions it was applied topically. The dye penetrated, stained, and stayed on the skin so long that it was applied for toenail rot and to treat planter warts. It was used for thrush (yeast infection), which transferred to the nipple during nursing; gentian violet was painted on a baby's mouth and a nursing mother's nipples as a precaution to prevent reinfection.

Gentian violet is a pert near permanent dye when applied to the skin. An English chemist named William Perkin originally synthesized aniline purple from coal tar as a dye. This breakthrough caught the attention of other chemists, and thus began the synthetic dye industry. In 1884, Hans Gram, a Danish physician, used aniline purple (gentian violet) as a component to develop the gram stain for identifying bacteria. Aniline purple was later replaced by crystal violet, methylrosaniline chloride (*United States Pharmacopoeia* XVI), which is a synthetic, more refined, easier-to-standardize form of the product. Gentian violet (crystal violet) still sees use today as a topical antibiotic in 1 percent aqueous or alcoholic solutions. Since water, heat, and light cause gentian violet to break down, solutions are best prepared fresh, kept in dark bottles away from heat, and used within a few months. Do not confuse gentian violet with gentian root, the plant, which was also used as a medicine. (60–p. 1100; 79–accessed October 21, 2002)

## GINGER (1100 A.D. TO DATE)

Ginger is the dried root (rhizome) of *Zingiber officinale*, family Zingiberaceae. There are many forms of ginger—African, Calcutta, Japanese, Martinique, and Jamaican. Its primary use as a medicinal was as a carminative, aromatic stimulant, and a flavoring for tonics. Ginger was a drug prone to adulteration in commerce with such ingredients or fillers as sawdust, flour, cereal products, and starches, which made it a "cheap" ingredient in whiskies and alcoholic beverages sold during the Prohibition era. Before enforcement authorities stepped in, as many as sixteen thousand persons died or suffered from paralysis due to drinking adulterated ginger liquors. Ginger was indeed, on occasion, a truly deadly additive, not so much on its own, as for the ingredients added to it by greedy businessmen to make a few bucks more.

Ginger contains gingerols, which have fever-reducing, pain-relieving, cough-suppressing, and antinausea properties. The oral dose of the dried root was 0.25 to 1 gram three times daily. A cup of tea made by steeping one gram in boiling water, steeping for ten to fifteen minutes, and then straining, was taken three times daily for morning sickness. (1–p. 278; 4–p. 475)

## GOLD (1595 TO DATE)

Gold has always been sought to fill man's hip pocket. Also known as aurum, "potable gold" was the resultant product of gold metal being placed in acid. Aurum was used to treat many early ailments. Its use was reported as early as 1595 to treat members of Queen Elizabeth's and Henry IV's courts. Today, it is still used in a 50 percent injectable solution (in the form of gold sodium thiomalate) as an antirheumatic (for arthritis) in the commercial preparations, myochrysine and aurolate, which are designed for intragluteal injection. Then and now, gold still gets man in the hip. (*Intragluteal* means deep in the biggest muscle of the butt.) (8–p. 322; 10)

## GOLDENROD AND JIMSON WEED

Yes, that's right, goldenrod and jimson, the weeds that grow wild in feedlots, were used as folk medicines. Goldenrod, *Solidago vigaurea, S. canadensis, and S. serotina*, family Asteraceae, were used interchangeably in tonics as a diuretic, for gouty arthritis and rheumatism, and to purify the blood. The powdered aboveground parts of the plant are classified as *aquaretrics* (agents that increase urine output without increasing sodium excretion). Taken with plenty of water, goldenrod was used for severe kidney and bladder pain. Its action was due to significant levels of saponins and flavonoids. A common dose was a cup of tea taken several times daily that was prepared by steeping a heaping teaspoonful of powdered plant in a half-a-stewer of water, letting set ten or so minutes, cooling, straining, then taking. A 1:1 liquid extract made from powder and whiskey was dosed at a half a teaspoonful.

Jimson weed, also called stink weed, *Datura stramonium*, family Solanaceae, was used to treat asthma, chest congestion, acute indigestion, and bad cough. *Bad cough* and *acute indigestion* were common frontiersmen's diagnoses, catchall phrases that covered a wide variety of ailments. Bad cough could mean anything from lung cancer to catarrhal bronchitis. Acute indigestion covered everything from pyrosis, chronic esophageal reflux, and stomach cancer to a heart attack.

"Say, whatever happened to old Jake Watson?"

"Aw, he up and died of acute indigestion from eating too much cantaloupe."

Or, "You know he died?"

"Git outta here."

"Yup. The bad cough finally got him."

The stems, seeds, and leaves of the jimson weed contain the potent and poisonous alkaloids atropine, hyoscyamine, and scopolamine. Concoctions made from the weed, in small amounts, slowed a cramping gut and helped control a bad case of "the running offs" (violent, watery diarrhea). The range between the therapeutic dose and toxic dose was much too narrow. An ill-prepared batch of jimson weed tea could just as easily cause a "fatal" case of acute indigestion as "cure" it, particularly in children. (4—p. 618)

## HOG LARD (1753–1960)

Medicinal hog lard was the processed fat obtained from the innards of butchered pigs. The crude fat was separated from muscle tissue and blood vessels, cut into pieces, and melted in wash pots and kettles. The liquid that rose to the top was skimmed off, strained through cheesecloth or course muslin, and allowed to harden. Pure hog lard was used as an emollient (a softening agent) that was soothing to the skin of particularly sensitive body parts. Its primary use was as a base for ointments, some of which contained powdered sulfur. The greasy yellow mixture was used for crotch rash (jock itch, male or female) and toe rot (athlete's foot). Hog lard, along with beeswax and pine resin, was a main ingredient in compound yellow basilicum, an ointment carried on the Lewis and Clark expedition. As with any animal product, hog lard readily rancified (spoiled) into a lumpy, oily mass that stunk like the soggy armpits of a cowboy who just spent a month in the saddle on a cattle drive. In warmer climates, it had to be sniffed good to determine if was still any good or not. (1; 4; 7)

## HONEYSUCKLE

Honeysuckle, also called goat's leaf and sweet vine, *Lonicera caprifolium* and *L. japonica*, family Caprifoliaceae, is a familiar vine to Texans. In bloom, its flowers have a sweet, characteristic, lemon-like odor, the odor of springtime in Texas. Whitetail deer particularly favor the vine's leaves and flowers as a food. Asian immigrants brought its use as a medicine to the Americas. The stems and flowers, prepared into infusions, were used for arthritis, as a diaphoretic, for bad colds, dysentery, and as an aperient. Externally, flower infusions were applied as washes for rashes and itching sores like poison ivy or for "acute itch" (topical allergies).

The flowers, leaves, and seed of the honeysuckle contain calcium, magnesium, tannins, saponins, and zinc. Modern evaluation suggests that medicinal preparations of honeysuckle have antibacterial activity against *Staph aureus*, *Salmonelli typhi*, tuberculosis-causing bacteria, influenza viruses, and even HIV. Data from modern animal studies suggest that honeysuckle is a central stimulant equivalent to nearly 20 percent of the activity of caffeine. Honeysuckle's high levels of saponins, particularly in the *L. japonica*, the Japanese honeysuckle, were so high that the immigrants used the plant to stun fish in ponds and slow-running streams. (4–p. 566; 80–accessed October 23, 2002)

## HORSETAIL

Also known as pewterwort (not peterwort), toadpipe, and scouring rush, horsetail (*Equisetum talmateia*, family Equisetaceae) has been used for ages to treat urinary problems—kidney stones, urinary tract irritations, and as a mild diuretic. Classically, the pulverized (powdered) stems were taken orally in teaspoonful doses, or brewed as a tea by boiling a heaping teaspoonful in a pint of water and drinking one cupful or taking one dose of the dry powder several times daily between meals. It was actually more effectively used as a wet compress on burns (ten grams of powder boiled in a liter of water). It has been reported to be helpful for everything from frostbite to halting profuse menstruation. The plant contains minute amounts of nicotine and flavone glycosides, active ingredients that reportedly break down vitamin B1. So, keep in mind that too much horsetail could make you weak. (4–575)

## ICHTHAMMOL

Ichthammol (sulfonated bitumen) was obtained by the destructive distillation of bituminous coal. Ichthammol ointment, better known as black drawing salve, was a mild irritant with astringent and antibacterial properties. Because of its drawing properties, mixed with camphor, sulfur, juniper tar, carbolic acid, and axle grease, ichthammol was a very popular remedy, which was used as a specific for treating boils (monstrous zits or pimples that developed on the body—a quite common ailment in frontier times). Topically it was (and still is) available in 10 and 20 percent ointments and as a product called Boil-Ease. (10–p. 633; 60–p. 724)

## IODINE

Iodine was prepared from the iodates in saltpeter by reduction with sulfites and from naturally occurring brines by oxidation with nitrites. Orally, iodine was used as an expectorant (it thinned thick mucous in the head, throat, and chest, making it easier to hack and spit up). Topically in 1 to 2 percent solutions, it was used as an antiseptic. Tinctures were notorious for staining the skin red. Added to water, iodine killed harmful bacteria that caused the runs (diarrhea). Iodine was often prepared in glycerin with carbolic acid (phenol) and used as a sore throat swab. Anyone who has ever had their throat swabbed with this concoction will never forget the medicinal smell, or taste, of phenol and iodine. A saturated solution of potassium iodide, SSKI, was a quite effective expectorant, which was used for years; but due to the more popular and much more stable synthetic product, guiafenesin, it has lost favor in medical practice. SSKI mixtures were unstable and had to be mixed fresh and stored in the refrigerator. Another salt of iodine, povidone iodide, is still used today. If you've had surgery recently and came back with a yellow belly, most likely they sterilized your abdomen with povidone iodide, which is sold under the trade name Betadine. (4–p. 598)

## IPECAC (1601 TO DATE)

The dried rhizomes and roots of ipecac, *Cephaelis ipecacuanha*, family Rubiaceae, often referred to the as "the creeping plant that makes you spit up," was a low-growing shrub that had wiry, reddish to dark brown roots. In small oral doses, it was used as an appetite stimulant and as an expectorant in croupy children. It was also used for dysentery. Its most common use was as an emetic to purge the system, particularly the stomach. Fifteen milliliters of ipecac syrup was enough to make even the meanest ol' fart in the valley get sick and throw up. An old James Bond movie comes to mind every time I think of ipecac. Bond wanted some information from an uncooperative associate, so he secretly doused the man's drink with ipecac. As they talked, Bond smiled and told the man he had given him a lethal dose of poison, and if he didn't tell him what he wanted, he wouldn't give him the antidote. The man laughed at first but when nausea set in, he spilled the beans, literally. Bond got his information, then laughed and said it was only ipecac and that he'd be all right in a few minutes.

Ipecac will make you throw up. The only problem is it makes you deathly-feeling sick in the process. Drinking several large glasses of water makes it work even faster. (1–p. 328; 4–p. 600)

## JALAP (1753 TO DATE)

The tuberous roots of jalap, *Convolvulus purga*, family Convolvulaceae, contain the glycosides, ipurganol, phytosterol, and jalapin, which were generally used as hydragogue, cathartics. A percolated mixture of the root, one part root, eight parts water, was allowed to stand; the resin that precipitated was collected and dried. A common dose was 125 milligrams of the resin. A tea was prepared by adding a teaspoonful of ground root to half of a small stewer of water, and sipped a cup at a time. Powdered root was dosed at three to twenty grains. The tincture was taken in two- to four-milliliter (half to one teaspoonfuls) doses. The pure resin was dosed at sixty to three hundred milligrams. (1–p. 260; 4–p. 608; 12–p. 143)

## JUNIPER TAR (1753–1955)

Juniper tar, also known as *Oleum juniperi* and prickly cedar, was the empyreumatic volatile oil obtained from the wood of the shrub, *Juniperus oxycedrus*, family Pinaceae. The woody parts of the plant were chopped, packed in containers with drains, and heated for several days. The tar that comes from the spigot separates itself into three layers. The oily upper layer was used in medicines. Topically it was used to treat eczema and psoriasis and to kill parasites (lice, ticks, etc.). (1–p. 234)

## KUDZU

*Pueraria lobata*, family Lubeminosae, is a malignant vine that grows on trees, fences, and hillsides, covering everything like an alien world. The parts used as medicine were the wiry roots, and the flowers. Orally, frontiersmen took three hundred milligrams of a root extract once daily for hangover and to help belay and quell the desire for, and effects of, too much whiskey. Chinese/Asian immigrants introduced kudzu's use as a medicinal to America. It is still used in China today. The active constituents of the plant are the isoflavones, daidzin, puerarin, and daidzein, which are thought to be reversible inhibitors of alcohol. Kudzu extract reportedly decreased alcohol consumption and peak alcohol levels, shortened alcohol-induced grogginess, and took the edge off alcohol cravings. Many "kick the habit" remedies for alcoholism the Army disease soldiers came home with were sold during and after the Civil War. Many contained little more than sugar, capsicum, and ipecac. The Asian remedies containing kudzu extract may have actually done some good. (4–p. 633)

## LICORICE-GLYCYRRHIZA (400 B.C. TO DATE)

The powdered roots of *Glycyrrhiza glabra*, family Fabaceae or Liguminaceae, was a perennial plant that grew to a height of three to five feet. The plant's roots contain a bitter principle known as glycyrrhizin, which is fifty times sweeter than cane sugar. Orally, the powdered root was used for chest and head inflammation, catarrh, cough, arthritis, and as a laxative. Combined with jalap, pinkroot, and cream of tarter, it was used for intestinal round worms. A typical dose was one to two tablespoonfuls every hour till worms expelled. Topically it was applied to the hair to reduce oiliness. A common dose of the powdered root was two to four grams. A tea was made by adding a level teaspoonful of powder to a cup of hot water, steeping ten minutes, straining, and drinking. (1–p. 158; 4–p. 666; 12–p. 143)

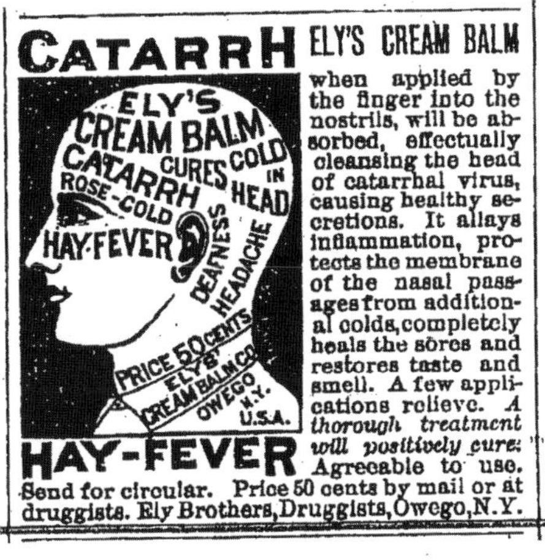


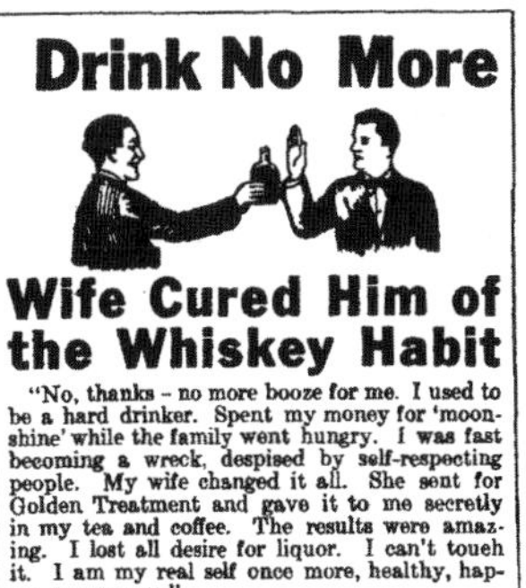


**Drink Habit Cured Secretly.**

**Trial Packages Mailed Free to Any One Sending Name and Address.**

After many years' trial Dr. J. W. Haines' discovery, Golden Specific, has received the hearty indorsement of such professional people as the Rev. Schimpfelman, the noted German divine; Dr. Rene Chabot, the world's greatest medical scientist; Franklyn Waters, the great

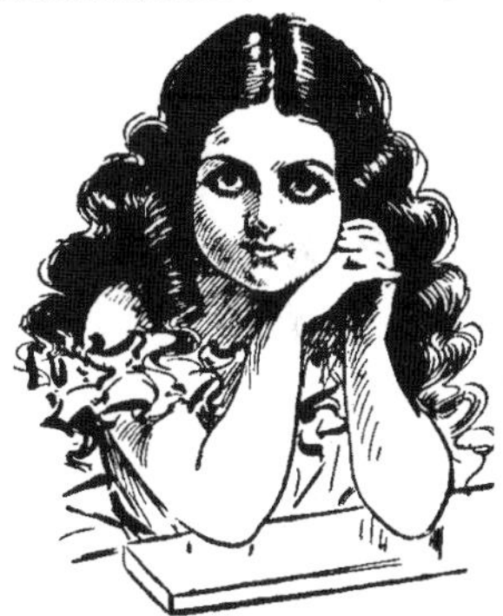

**A Little Girl Who Quickly Cured Her Papa Who Was an Awful Drunkard Without His Knowledge.**

temperance lecturer, and hundreds of others. Golden Specific is odorless and tasteless, is mixed with coffee, tea, milk or food and given the drunkard secretly. Its effect is remarkable, caring cases that seemed absolutely hopeless.

Send your name and address to Dr. J. W. Haines, 1,614 Glenn Building, Cincinnati, Ohio, and he will mail a free trial package of the remedy to you securely sealed in a plain wrapper, also full directions how to use it, books and testimonials from hundreds who have been cured and everything needed to aid you in saving those near and dear to you from a life of degradation and ultimate poverty and disgrace.

## MANURE

Yes, manure, cow dung, plain old bullshit tea, is mentioned in an early folk medicine manual as a medical treatment. The dried chips were reportedly steeped in boiling water and taken orally to treat consumption. *Consumption*, in pioneer days, was a catchall term for many undetermined illnesses, most of which were later determined to be tuberculosis. Families in Tennessee that raised sheep made "sheep tea" from sheep dung, which reportedly made measles break out in children. They gave them a glass and covered them with heavy blankets till the breakout was complete.

Grandma Leorah told me that her grandmother used to mix powdered cow manure with water and added done-been-chewed-once tobacco that was still wet. The gritty poultice was applied to wasp stings and insect bites. Boy, talk about using what you got plenty of on a farm.

Grandma never made a bull manure/tobacco poultice for my brothers or me when we got wasp stung. She simply dug a finger into her bottom lip and smeared wet snuff on the sting. As I remember, the gooey mess worked. At least I thought it did. Her holding me close, rocking, and giving me the old "poor baby" treatment might have had something to do with my feeling better. (11–p. 16)

## MAYAPPLE (1820 TO DATE)

Also known as mandrake or podophyllium, mayapple consists of the dried roots of a plant in the Berberidaceae family. The plant was a perennial herb that grew in Virginia and North Carolina. Indians introduced mayapple to early settlers.

Podophyllum resin (1863 to date) is a refined powdered mixture prepared from dried mayapple roots by a percolation process using acidified water. The powdered and dried resin has a "snuffy" odor and is a caustic (destroys organic tissue by chemical degradation). That means it burned like hell if dabbed on anything other than affected tissues. Applied topically it was used to treat certain papillomas. Taken orally, it is a hydragogue cathartic. Hydragogue refers to the process of taking on huge amounts of water. The purgative dose of podophyllum resin was ten milligrams.

Papilloma, papilloma. Hydrogogue, hydrogogue. Don't you just love these words? They sound so . . . pappy and goggy.

If you don't think pioneers had yucky problems, listen to this. Papillomas are branching or lobelike, benign tumors. Uterine cervix papillomas occur as small, red lesions that project from above surrounding vaginal mucosa and resemble a cockscomb. Penile papillomas occur as wartlike, pearly elevations of skin on the edge of the penis. Was it not an astounding discovery when, a few days after a barn dance, you look in your britches and find something like that?

A hydragogue cathartic not only purged the gut, it did it voluminously (I love that word, too) and, oftentimes, explosively. You don't reckon this is where, in frontier times, the old pot beside the bed got its stormy name, do you? (1; 4; 9)

## MERCURY (3000 B.C. TO DATE)

It is interesting to note in many old pictures taken of our forefathers, just how many pioneer women had caged canaries as pets. Originally, the birds were brought west as gas detectors in mercury and silver mines. Odorless gases that were formed during the mining processes killed many miners. Canaries were supersensitive to the poisonous gases. The birds were carried in cages into the mine; when a bird fell over dead, the miners evacuated that shaft until it could be properly ventilated. The little bird's beautiful songs were no doubt a welcomed relief to lonely pioneer women, particularly during those periods of heavy silence after an endless night with a sick or dying child.

Mild mercurous chloride, also known as calomel (1753 to date), was obtained by sublimating the product of a trituration of mercuric sulfate, quicksilver, and sodium chloride in boiling water. It was a heavy yellowish white, tasteless product that was used as a stimulant, cathartic, and antibacterial for practically every disease imaginable. Taken orally, the toxic effects of calomel produced fetid breath, spongy gums, sensitive teeth, salivation, muscle trembling, and general weakness. Its most popular uses were in the treatment of syphilis (as an antimicrobial) and to purge the system of all the "bad stuff" that had gotten in it (a cholagogue, liver stimulant, and cathartic). Mercury was a true deadly elixir. For venereal diseases it was dosed until the symptoms of poisoning (fetid breath and bleeding gums, etc.) appeared. Its action against syphilis was specific and well proven. However, the therapeutic ranges varied so that many times it was hard to determine whether the mercury did the permanent damage, or the condition. Most frontier health professionals attributed any debilitation (brain damage) to the disease rather than the cure.

Inhalations in the form of the vapor of mercury were administered as a treatment for membranous croup, venereal disease ulcerations of the mouth and throat, and diphtheria.

The most commonly used preparations were these:

- *Pills* (often called blue mass pills, which contained mercury, honey, rose water, licorice root, and rose petals) and compound cathartic pills, the dose being two or three of the three-grain doses. They were used for biliousness, depression, and dysenteric diarrhea.
- *Gray powders* that were made from mercury and chalk, the dose for children being from a half to five grains, were used for acute indigestion and vomiting.
- *Blue ointment and plasters* (in liver pads) were applied over enlarged glands, chronically inflamed joints, and goiters.
- *Calomel* (mild mercurous chloride), the most common oral dosage being from five to fifteen grains, was used as a cathartic.
- *Corrosive sublimate* (strong mercurous chloride), the most dangerous and toxic, was used as a cathartic and for treating

syphilis. It was dosed at from one one-hundredth to one-sixteenth of a grain.

- *Yellow wash*, which was made from corrosive sublimate and limewater (one dram of drug to a pint of limewater), was used as a stimulating application to old venereal ulcers and as a penis flush.
- *Black wash*, made of calomel and lime-water (one dram/pint of lime-water), was used to remove venereal warts then dusting with powdered calomel.

Calomel use pretty much died in the early part of the twentieth century and is no longer used. The external mercurial, Thiomersol (a tincture/solution containing 49 percent mercury) is still used today for antisepsis of the skin prior to surgery and for first aid treatment. (10–p. 635; 18–pp. 1099–100; 61–pp. 474–75; 68–accessed September 29, 2002)

## MESQUITE

The bark, sap, leaves, and seeds of the shrubby tree *Prosopis glandulosa*, *P. pubescens*, and *P. velutina*, family Fabaceae—also known, respectively, as the honey mesquite, the screwbean mesquite, and the velvet pod—were a significant food source. The lowly Texas coyote in late summer consumed the beans of the tree as a means of survival. Native Texas Americans have long relied on the mesquite pod as a medicinal staple from which they made tea, syrup, and a type of flour or ground meal they called *pinole*. Mesquite bark was used to make baskets and clothing fabric. The wood and roots were used as fuel. A concoction made by bruising the leaves in water was applied as an astringent to sore eyes. A tea tonic was prepared from the bark. Made into poultices, the beans were used as a soothing relief for sunburn and insect bites. The comforting, demulcent activity of mesquite was due to high concentrations of a natural gum it contained. Early druggists used mesquite gum as a binding agent in pill making. (83–accessed November 2003, March 2002)

## MILK

Yes, cow's milk was used as a medicine. It even appeared in the official compendium, the National Formulary from 1916 to 1942. In earlier times, the French claimed that buttermilk was invaluable as the lactic acid in it dissolves and prevents ossification (thickening of the tissues) of heart valves, arteries, and soft-tissue cartilages. Raw cow's milk, well sweetened, combined with senna, Carolina pinkroot, American worm seed, and manna, was touted as a "cure" for intestinal roundworms. Unboiled raw cow's milk was used for diarrhea, stomachache, and dysentery. (1–p. 59; 12–61; 12–p. 108)

## MILK THISTLE

The aboveground parts of plain old milk thistle, *Silybum marianum*, family Asteraceae, was used to maintain health by stimulating the gallbladder, for treating jaundice, pleurisy, malaria complaints, and improving menstrual flow. The plant was grown in Europe as a vegetable and as a spinach substitute, which was used in salads. The white exudates that oozed from the broken plant was applied to burns, to ant bites, and to bull nettle stings. The dried seeds of the milk thistle were ground and used by early American pioneers as a substitute for coffee. (4–732)

## NUTGALL (450 B.C. TO 1955)

You know them little balls that grow on oak trees that look like acorns but ain't? Well, they're called *galls*. An insect called *Cynips tinctoria* punctures a young oak tree's stem and lays her eggs inside the tender bark. This causes an irritation and what is called an *excrescence*, which is an unnatural growth of the tree's limb. As the larvae begin to develop inside this round, nut-looking ball, it enlarges and can reach the size of a full-grown acorn or bigger. Texas nutgall is what's inside these nutty growths. Toward the end of July, the bug matures, drills a hole, and leaves. The best nutgall was gathered during the middle of July while the insect was still inside. The galls were pulverized and dried and dissolved in water or alcohol. Taken orally, it was used to treat dysentery and bloody diarrhea. Gargled, it was used for ulcers caused by taking too much mercury. Mixed with milk, it was used for diarrhea in children. Applied locally as a tincture, it was used as an astringent. Adding alum to gall in a water-based decoction was used to heal burns. The active ingredient in gall was tannic acid. Texas nutgalls yield up to 40 percent tannic acid, which made them a convenient source of tannic acid to tan hides. A common oral dose of powdered gall was five to twenty grains; of an infusion, one or two tablespoonfuls; of a tincture, one dram. Dosed at one gram, Texas nutgall was also used as an antidote for strychnine and for poisonings from overdoses of digitalis and other vegetable alkaloids. (1–p. 174; 78–accessed October 20, 2002)

## NUX VOMICA (1640–1989)

Nux vomica was the dried ripe seed of the tree, *Strychnos nux vomica*, family Loganiaceae. The fruit was a berry that had a bitter pulp. As a poison for animals, it was used in Europe during the sixteenth century. Nux vomica contains the alkaloids strychnine, brucine, and igasurine. Nux vomica was classed as a bitter and was used for its "stimulant" properties. Mixed as a tincture with cantharides and tincture of iron and quinine, it was used for impotency. A common oral dose was a hundred milligrams. An overdose began with twitching muscles, then tonic and clonic muscle spasms, delirium, and death. No topical preparations were found. (1–p. 348; 4–p. 766; 12–pp. 48, 183)

## OAK BARK (1753 TO DATE)

The powdered bark of the common oak tree, *Quercus robur*, *Q. petraea*, and *Q. alba*, family Fagaceae, was prepared in teas by steeping a gram of coarsely ground bark in boiling water, steeping, straining, and drinking. It was taken for diarrhea, colds, fever, and as a stomachic. As a topical, it was used for oral rinses, on wet compresses, in poultices, for inflammation, sore throat, chilblains, and as a soothing soak for rectal and vaginal gaulding, and to stop bleeding. (4–p. 767)

## OLIVE OIL (1753 TO DATE)

Also called sweet oil, olive oil is the fixed oil obtained from the ripe fruit of *Olea europeae*, family Oleaceae, a small evergreen tree that grows in Mediterranean countries. In frontier times, it was imported but later was cultivated in subtropical localities. Olive oil consists chiefly of olien. Warm olive oil instilled into the ear not only softened earwax but helped with pain. Orally, it was taken as a demulcent laxative. (1–p. 183; 4–p. 777)

## ONION (1753 TO DATE)

*Allium cepa*, family Alliaceae, the common onion, was used as an anthelmintic, to stop cough, bronchitis, and for asthma, dehydration, and as a menstruation aid. Combined with tobacco leaves, onion was layered and placed on hot coals until soft and applied to bruises. The warm juice was also squeezed and allowed to drop in the ear. This remedy reportedly gave immediate relief for earache. (4–p. 779; 12–p. 77)

## OPIUM, LAUDANUM, MORPHINE, AND CODEINE

Opium (700 B.C. to date) was the air-dried milky exudates obtained from incising unripe pods of *Papaver somniferum*, family

Papaveraceae. Dioscorides, in the second century, was the first to write about a potion called diacodion, which was a syrup made from poppies. The active constituent of diacodion (opium) was morphine (1817 to date), which was discovered by a German named Frederick Serturner who presented his findings to the world in a paper in 1817. As a result of a British victory over the Chinese (the Anglo-Chinese war of 1856), opium's use was legalized. The British had begun to take over the drug's trade as early as 1833. After the war, opium became an even more significant source of revenue for Britain. With domination of the market, a very lucrative and addictive drug trade began. Thomas De Quincey, a famous opium eater and addict, actually consumed a mixture of opium and alcohol known as laudanum.

In the sixteenth century, Paracelsus introduced laudanum (sixteenth century to date) to Western cultures where, in the nineteenth century, it became a "proper and well-accepted medicine" used for everything from sleeplessness to consumption. To prepare laudanum, they dissolved as much opium in a jug of whiskey or moonshine as possible.

Opium had a very offensive, snuffy, and bitter taste. Suspending it in alcohol made it even worse. The main advantage of putting opium in whiskey was that the alcohol dissolved the narcotic constituents of the plant so it was more readily absorbed; and too, alcohol acted like a preservative to keep the opium "actively" fresh. Laudanum was little more than a crude tincture of opium. Each lot varied in strength with the alcohol and form of drug used.

Most laudanum contained the equivalent of ten grams of powdered or gum opium in four ounces of 80 proof liquor (the standard 40 to 50 percent content of most rotgut whiskies of the period). The dose of this concentration was fifteen to twenty drops, which was less than one milliliter, or roughly a quarter of a teaspoonful. Most laudanum was sold in dropper bottles and dosed by the dropper or fractions thereof depending on its delivery volume.

The famous poet Elizabeth Barrett Browning and the famous author Charles Dickens were but a few of the slaves to the nectar of the poppy. Much of their poetic and creative inspiration came from laudanum.

Paregoric (1715 to date), also known as *Camphorae composita tinctura*, *Tinctura opii benzoica*, and *Paregoricum elixir* in British pharmacopoeias, was a camphorated opium tincture prepared by the cold maceration of powdered opium (4.3 grams), anise oil (3.8 milliliters), benzoic acid (3.8 grams), and camphor (3.8 grams) for five days, occasionally shaking, in diluted alcohol (nine hundred milliliters) and glycerin (thirty-eight milliliters). The resulting concoction was filtered and enough alcohol added to make the volume total 950 milliliters. Paregoric was (and still is) used for diarrhea, stomach cramps, and cough. The usual dose is one to two teaspoonfuls four times daily. Paregoric has a bittersweet, licorice-like odor and taste. In frontier times, it was a popular sugartit additive for colic in babies. For years, it could be bought without a prescription (over the counter), but its abuse potential became such a problem, it was finally placed on prescription-only status in Texas. It is seldom used today but still available.

Codeine (1832 to date) was isolated from opium in 1832 by a Frenchman named Robiquet. The problem was that there was such a small amount of the codeine in opium that it didn't become popular as a medicinal agent until the process of methylating morphine was developed. For years it was viewed as a weak morphine. Besides, in frontier times, opium was cheaper and more readily available. Codeine had the advantage that it was less apt to cause nausea, vomiting, and constipation, but these benefits were not expanded upon until well into the twentieth century. Today, because of these advantages and a considerable less amount of paperwork involved in dispensing it, more codeine is used in the retail prescription trade than morphine. (60–p. 1044–46)

Cocaine (1882 to date) was the dried leaves of *Erythroxylon coca*, family Erythroxylaceae. An alkaloid obtained from the leaves by extraction with dilute acid was purified, then crystallized. Cocaine was used as a topical anesthetic. It is still used today for patients allergic to modern anesthetics. (1–p. 315)

## PEPPERMINT (400 B.C. TO DATE)

*Menthae piperitae*, family Labiatae, consisted of the dried leaf and flowering tops of the plant. The perennial was indigenous to Europe but was naturalized in the United States. The dried and pulverized leaves were used as a stomachic, for acute indigestion, and for morning sickness. The oil distilled from the plant's stems was rectified by distillation. A common dose of the oil was 0.1 milliliter.

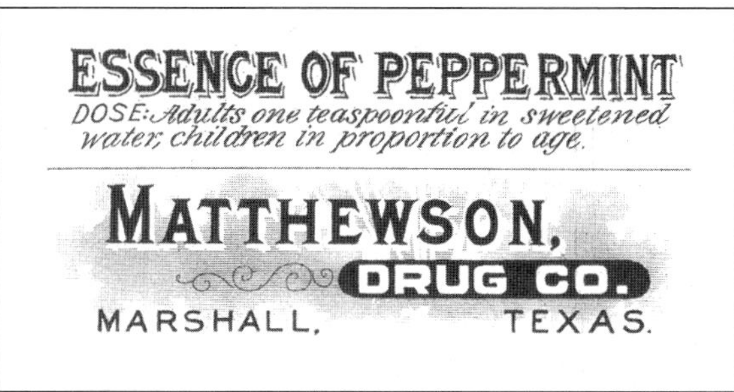


The medicinally active ingredients in peppermint were menthol (50 to 78 percent), acetaldehyde, acetic acid, and valeric acid. It was applied topically as a counterirritant and used as a flavoring for candies and chewing gum. (1–p. 205; 4–p. 819; 12–p. 108)

## PERSIMMON

The unripe fruit of *Diospyros virginiana*, family Ebenaceae, plain old persimmon, was mashed, deseeded, and applied as an astringent. The lip-puckering juice of green persimmon contains tannins and malic acid as active ingredients. It was used topically as a styptic and taken internally as an emetic. Green persimmon juice was so bitter, if you didn't puke, you darned sure got better, just so you didn't have to take another dose. As an officially recognized medicinal, green persimmon was listed in official compendiums (the *United States Pharmacopoeia*) only from 1820 to 1882. (1–p. 175)

## PERUVIAN BARK (1753–1955)

Also known as cinchona, cinchonia bark, and calisaya, Peruvian bark was the pulverized, dried bark (roots and stems) of six- to nine-year-old *Cinchona succirubra* trees (a type of evergreen). Other known hybrids of the tree were yellow cinchona, calisaya bark, yellow bark, and red cinchona. The active ingredient of Peruvian bark, quinine (pioneer aspirin), wasn't extracted from the bark until 1845. Lewis and Clark carried on their expedition in 1803 fifteen pounds of Peruvian bark (one-third of their total dollar expenditure for medicinals).

Early missionaries learned about the plant from Indians in Peru who, overcome with fever, drank water from a pond laden with fallen cinchona trees and were cured of their ills and chills.

The drug itself helped make exploration and settling of the west possible. Peruvian bark was used to treat fever, chills, and ague (malaria). It was used as a bitter in tonics to aid digestion and restore muscle tone. Mixed with gunpowder into a poultice, it was used to treat gunshot wounds and snakebites. It was formally given orally in one-gram (sixty-grain) doses (that's about a quarter of a teaspoonful). (1; 4; 7)

## PINE (1753 TO DATE)

All parts of the pine tree—the wood, the bark, the needles, and sprouts—were used to make frontier medicines. Pine bark was first official in the *National Formulary* in 1916; pine oil, 1947. Pine needle oil was officially recognized as a medicine in the *United States Pharmacopoeia* from 1916 to 1947 and in the *National Formulary* from 1947 to date. Pine oil was listed in Lewis's *Edinburg New Dispensary* in 1753.

The sprouts of the pine were used for catarrh, respiratory complaints, bad cold, congestion, and hoarseness. Pine oil was extracted by fractionation and steam distillation of pine sawdust, a profitable by-product of sawmills. The oil contains terpineol, terpenes, phenolic ethers, and methyl chavicol as active ingredients. It was used as a disinfectant and insecticide. Orally it helped cut phlegm from the throat (the hacky crud as my grandpa called it). The outer corky layer of the bark was removed and separated and extracted with alcohol. The resultant product was used by early druggist to prepare syrup bases for medications—two common products were cosadein and prunicodeine. Common doses of the sprout were two to nine grams. A tea made by boiling the same amount in a cup of water and taken was also used. A few drops of pine needle oil dropped into a stewer of boiling water and inhaled was used for congestion and for bronchitis. Pine oil was used in cough drops and as flavoring in chewable laxative tablets. Topically it was applied in 20 to 50 percent alcoholic extracts and applied or added to baths. (1–pp. 214, 248, 283; 4–836; 60–pp. 725, 1235)

## PINKROOT (1820–1926)

Also known as American wormgrass, the roots of *Spigelia marilandica*, family Loganiaceae, contained a volatile alkaloid, spigeline, a bitter, nicotine-like product that was used to treat worms. The plant was a perennial indigenous to the southern United States. Pinkroot roots were dried, crushed, and pulverized. Dosed at half to one level teaspoonful twice daily, or prepared into a tea by adding two teaspoonfuls to a quart of boiling water, cooling, straining, and taking two wineglasses per day, it made an excellent "dewormer" for both pinworms and roundworms. Infusions of pinkroot were commonly combined with strong laxatives or cathartics to aid in worm removal. Pinkroot liquid preparations were notorious for staining clothing red. (4–837; 18–p. 1103)

## POKEWEED (1820–1947)

The root of *Phytolacca americana*, family Phytolaccaceae, was ground and taken orally as an emetic. Frontiersmen used the ground root and crushed berries for rheumatism and skin infections (ringworm, scabies, etc).

All parts of the poke plant, save for the leaves in the spring, are potently poison. Boiled and poured off two or three times, the leaves, known to us country folks as "polk salad," is a delightful substitute for fresh spinach or turnip greens.

## POMEGRANATE (1753–1936)

Pomegranate as a medicine was derived from the plant *Punica granatum*, family Punicaceae. The active constituents of all parts of the plant were tannins. The anthelmintic (worm-killing ability) wasn't discovered until 1878 when the active ingredient pelletierine, a combination of four alkaloids, was isolated. The dried plant parts were ground and mixed with lime and extracted with chloroform. The extract was used in combination with other remedies (pumpkin seeds and croton oil) as a taenifuge (expelled tapeworms) and a vermifuge (expelled worms and intestinal parasites). (1–p. 299; 12–p. 145)

## POND LILY

Native Americans and pioneers used the water lily, *Nympheae odorata*, better known as the American white pond lily, as a medicine. Though it never achieved status in official compendiums, as a folk medicine it was used with quite good results. In poultices, it was applied to the throat and mouth for irritations, and as a soothing agent for burns and abrasions like saddle sores, on both horse and man. The root, the medicinal part of the plant, contains tannins, which are responsible for its antiseptic and astringent properties. Taken orally, a tea was prepared by steeping a teaspoonful of the ground root in a cup of boiling water, straining, letting cool, and sipping it to ease a sore throat and for diarrhea. Liquid extracts (one gram of powdered root to one ounce of whiskey) were prepared and dosed at a teaspoonful several times a day as needed.

Women of repute (and ill repute) used the concoctions as douches. During a time when people used whatever medicinal they had access to, soothing hot poultices prepared from the water lily's roots were applied for practically every topical irritation known to early westerners. (4–p. 57; 76–accessed October 18, 2002)

## POTASH

Campfire and fireplace ashes have been used in medicines for time on end. Lye soap, the homemade cleaning bar, was as common to the pioneer as beans and fried taters. Lye was obtained by first filling a barrel about a fourth full with straw or hay, packing it, and then adding wood ashes. A hole drilled in the side of the barrel at the bottom was corked. Water was slowly poured over the ashes, allowed to sit a minute, and then the cork was removed allowing the brackish liquid to flow into an appropriate container. This liquid was a crude form of potassium hydroxide, better known as potash water or lye water, and was used itself as a caustic or a blistering agent for pain. In weaker solutions it was used to stop bleeding.

Making soap was a simple process. Eight to ten pounds of clean hog lard was melted in a huge pot, two quarts of water were added, and two cups of the solution obtained from the ash barrel. The mixture was boiled a couple hours with occasional stirring (additional water added if needed), removed from the fire, and poured into molds or pans to be cut into squares. The congealed solid was lye soap. Adding pine oil or other antiseptic oils while it boiled not only made the soap smell better but made it antiseptic, too. (60–p. 727; 81–accessed October 31, 2002)

## PRICKLY PEAR CACTUS

Also known as cactus flower and Indian fig, the prickly pear's medicinal parts are the spiny leaves, flowers, and fruit of *Opuntia streptacantha* and *Phaecantha*, family Cataceae. Taken orally in teas, cooked, or in dried extracts, the young lobes were used to treat diabetes. The flowers when taken orally were used for colic, diarrhea, and prostate problems. When ripe, the fruit is still used to make jellies and candies.

The young lobes were and still are consumed today as a delicacy. Eating cactus will reduce blood sugar. Its mechanism of action lies in its pectin content. Pectin is known to alter liver metabolism of cholesterol. The problem comes in dosing. If one consumes enough cacti to cause a significant lowering of blood sugar, it becomes toxic to the kidneys. Frontiersmen didn't know that. All they knew was that they felt better after eating it. The backache they got later was simply attributed to something else.

Now don't go out and try to bite a ripe prickly pear just to see what it taste like. Believe me, they suck. But if you're like me and you just gotta do it anyway to prove how terrible it tastes, please, singe off the stickers first. A friend of mine read a magazine article about making jelly out of ripe prickly pears. The idea amused him so, on a backpacking trip, he boldly plucked a ripe pear and bit into it. His lips were swollen like an old milk cow's for weeks. Took him a month to tweezer all them stickers out of his fingers, too. Now you might say to yourself that no one in his right mind, save for an imbecile, would do something like that. Well, my friend did. And he ain't no imbecile— he's a physician, a specialist, and a darned good one at that.

Indian legend had it that a hair must be plucked from a gatherer's head so the cactus would yield pears that wouldn't twist the heart and mind. Spirit worship was common among Indian tribes. A gatherer dared to risk offending the spirits.

Prickly pears are high in calcium and are very mucilaginous. Eating them acted like an antacid. Here is an old recipe I discovered on how to prepare prickly pear jelly. I haven't tried it yet, but I will give copy of it to my doctor friend.

**Prickly Pear Jelly**

3 cups prickly pear juice prepared by mashing and straining red-ripe fruits, the more juice the better.
2 tablespoons lemon juice
3 cups sugar
2 tablespoons commercial canning pectin (Sure Jell, I think it's called.)

Mix juice and pectin preparation, bring to fast boil, and add lemon juice; add water as needed to keep it thick but liquid. Stir in sugar, boil three to four minutes, skim off foam, and place in sterilized jars. Cover with hot paraffin and seal.

The famous Texas Ranger, Bigfoot Wallace, after a battle with the Comanches in 1874 reportedly applied a cactus remedy, which he said was the best wound medicine he had ever tried. The preparation he used was made by the Morley Brothers Drug Company in Austin. The company guaranteed their cactus line products with a money-back guarantee. Their miraculous salves were recommended for everything from boils, burns, bites, and bruises, to colds, molds, and sore tail holes. (39–p. 15; 83–accessed November 3, 2002)

## ROCK CANDY

Rock candy, pure, crystallized sugar, has been used for centuries. Recognized as having marked therapeutic and preservative qualities, in frontier times it was used only as a medicine or preservative clear up to the middle of the eighteenth century. The earliest known date it was recorded was somewhere around the middle of the 1200s. In 1584, an English reference cites the medicinal value of the "Sugre Candie." In 1596, Shakespeare mentioned its therapeutic value as a throat soother for long-winded talkers.

The gospel according to Leorah gives me my best experience with rock candy. She called her concoction a hot toddie. Her warm dose of medicine contained rock candy, lemon juice, and good old moonshine that Grandpa and Old Tub used to sit on the porch and drink. In lieu of lemon, sometimes she shook in a squirt of vanilla flavoring. The warm liquid tasted weirdly wonderful and did seem to help a sore throat. Sometimes I was even guilty of faking a raw hack just to get her to give me another dose.

## SAGE (1753–1950)

Also known as salvia, sage is the dried leaf of *Salvia officinalis*, family Labiatae. In Latin, *salvia* means "salve." The herb is a perennial that grows to a height of less than two feet. The leaves were gathered while still flowering and carefully dried in the shade. It has an odor likened to that of lavender and was used as a condiment, as a perfume, and to help preserve meat. Taken orally, it acted as a stimulant, carminative, and stomachic. Common sage was also known as German sarsaparilla.

Sage contains volatile oils composed of camphor and thujone, which have antiflatulent, antibacterial, fungicidal, and antiperspirant properties. Sage leaves were also an excellent source of beta-carotene. Sage has anhidrotic activity (stops or slows perspiration). A decoction of sage (boiled water extract) was used to help dry a mother's milk and to relieve the hot sweats of menses. The toxic properties of thujone when taken orally (convulsions and mental deterioration) were sage's medicinal downfall.

The use of muscatel sage (from the plant *Salvia sclarea*, family Labiatae/Lamiaceae) came to us from Europe. Also called clary sage, muscatel sage was used as a stomachic and for digestive disorders. Topically, the mucilage obtained from sage was used to help remove foreign objects from the eye. The principal means of action was the same as the mucilage on flaxseeds. The expressed oils from sage were used in perfumes, as flavoring agents, and in frontier cosmetics. An antiperspirant product called Salvysat is still currently marketed in Germany. (1–p. 208; 4–pp. 290, 923; 67–p. 271)

## SARSAPARILLA (1500 TO DATE)

The sarsaparilla used in the old west came primarily from Mexico and Central America. The name *Zarza para illa* was Spanish, meaning "a small, twisting vine." Zarzaparilla was, and still is, prepared from the orange hued roots of the *Smilax linné* plant (family Liliaceae).

Sarsaparilla's use dates back to the early sixteenth century. The Chinese called it *tu fu ling* and used it to treat venereal disease and as an aphrodisiac. The sarsaparilla preparations consumed by American cowboys were thought to make them more virile and help ward off the nasty head colds their privates got after going to brothels. Sarsaparilla drinks *were* diuretic in action and *did* act as alterative tonics to cleanse the urinary tract. The drinks were also touted to help relieve aching backs and the sore butt bones (arthritis and rheumatism) pursuant to spending long stretches in the saddle. (1–p. 130; 12–p. 204)

## SASSAFRAS (1512 TO DATE)

Also referred to as saxifrax or sassafrax by salty Texas pioneers with a "jaw fulla chaw," *Sassafras ablidum*, family Lauraceae, was the dried bark root of a tree indigenous to the south. Seminole Indians used sassafras as a medicine long before Ponce de Leon made his famous landing in Florida. Orally, sassafras was used for urinary tract problems, throat inflammation, syphilis, and as a blood purifier. The active ingredient in sassafras was safrole, a volatile oil that was used to flavor early root beer drinks. A tea made from a half a teaspoonful of ground root to a mug of boiling water, steeped, and strained, was taken for catarrh, arthritis, kidney disorders. Topically, a paste made with kerosene or turpentine was applied to rashes and used to treat "white skin rot" (skin cancers) and old age spots. The most popular use of sassafras today is as a sprinkle additive to gumbos, which is called *filé* (pronounced "fee-lay"). (1–p. 240; 4–p. 933)

## SENNA (400 B.C. TO DATE)

*Senna alexandrina*, family Leguminosae, consists of the dried leaves and bark of the low growing bush. Senna contains several sennosides, which have laxative and cathartic action, depending on the dose, when taken orally. Prepared in teas by soaking two heaping teaspoonfuls in a cup of warm water, when taken at bedtime, made getting up in the morning a rather urgent matter. Senna is one of the more gentle medicines frontiersmen took to help "clean them out." It is still used today as the product Senokot in many hospitals as the drug of choice to help "move" Mama after she's had a baby. (4–p. 942; 10–p. 319)

## SLIPPERY ELM (1753 TO DATE)

Also known as Indian elm or sweet elm, the inner bark of the slippery elm, *Ulmus rubra* and *fulva*, family Ulmaceae, was used for sore throat. It was contained in many oral lozenges for its ability to sooth mucous membranes and upper gut problems. It was used in some old remedies for expelling tapeworms. It was also consumed to relieve the pain of what we today call reflux, that hindering burning in the lower throat from stomach acid that seeps up the esophagus from the stomach. Topically it was applied to burns, cold sores, boils, and abscesses. Slippery elm worked because it provided a steady release of mucilage, which coated, soothed, and protected the linings of the throat and upper gut. You might say it was a frontiersman's version of today's sulcrafate (the trademarked product known as Carafate).

## SNAKEROOT (1753 TO DATE)

Texas snakeroot, *Aristolochia reticulata*, family Aristolochiaceae, was a twining vine that wove its way over and through surrounding foliage in Texas, Louisiana, Arkansas, and Oklahoma woodlots. The roots were collected and dried and used to treat snakebite, fever, insanity, constipation, rheumatism, and what was called "fits" (epilepsy). The active ingredient in snakeroot was borneol and serpentarin, which were good for a condition called "red face and ears," as Grandma Leorah called it. This was a flushing state exhibited by patients with high blood pressure. Snakeroot was used as a stimulant in many bitters, which were sold during the late nineteenth and early twentieth centuries. (1–p. 211; 4–p. 592)

## STINGING NETTLE (1753 TO DATE)

Stinging nettle, common nettle, or bull nettle as we call it in Texas (see "Urea") is a plant, *Urtica dioica*, family Urticaceae. Orally, prepared as a tea by steeping a heaping teaspoonful of the ground plant parts in a gill (eight tablespoonfuls or a half a cup) of boiling water and straining it, it was used for inflammation and infection of the kidney and bladder. Raw nettle juice was used as an analgesic.

Topically, it was used for rheumatism by preparing it in a 25 percent alcohol tincture. Bull nettle flowers in early summer to produce a nutlike fruit about the size and with the same color markings as a huge tick just before it drops from a dog's ear. The nuts are tasty, quite similar to that of a ripe chinquapin (pronounced "chinky-pin"). If you don't know what a chinquapin tastes like, you just ain't lived much at all.

## SULFUR (1753 TO DATE)

Burned in an enclosed room and inhaled, sulfur was used to treat scarlet fever; to disinfect ships and buildings of plague-carrying fleas; and used in axle grease as an antiseptic. (12–p. 61)

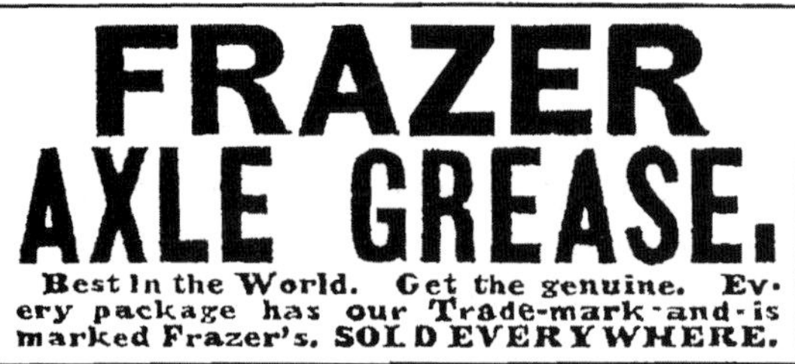


## TICKLE TONGUE (1820 TO DATE)

The tickle tongue tree, often referred to by older Texans as "the toothache tree," *Zanthoxylum hirsutum*, and *Z. americanum*, family Rutaceae, is also known as prickly ash because of its spiny, sticker-infested bark. The berry and the bark are the medicinal parts of the tree. The name tickle tongue comes from the numbing, almost-effervescent feeling one gets when applying the moist, inner layer of freshly removed bark to the tongue. Tickle tongue was used by frontiersmen to treat stomach cramps, as a tonic, as a stimulant, and for toothache. Tickle tongue bark and berries contain as active ingredients, nitidine, chelerythrine, asarinin, and neoherculin, which have anti-inflammatory, antibiotic, antitubercular, and stimulant properties. In large doses, these ingredients can be toxic. Prepared in tonics, it was used for "weak legs," a medical condition known today as intermittent claudication (sporadic spells of slowed circulation). A common dose of the dried, powdered bark was two grams (half a teaspoonful). A tea was made by boiling two grams of dried bark in a cup of boiling water, steeping fifteen minutes, and then straining. A 1:1 alcoholic extract was dosed at two milliliters three times daily. A tincture of one part powdered bark and five parts whiskey was dosed at a half to one teaspoonful three times daily. Tickle tongue berries were dried and powdered and taken in one-gram doses; a 1:1 extract made with whiskey was dosed at 0.5 to 1.5 milliliters. Tickle tongue and burdock were active ingredients in the famous Hoxsey Cancer Formula (discussed earlier). (1–p. 269; 4–p. 763, 971; 81–accessed October 24, 2002)

## TOLU (1574 TO DATE)

Tolu is a balsam extracted from *Myroxylon balsamum*, family Lequminosae, by cutting grooves (the same as turpentining only using several long, narrow, V-like cuts in the bark and catching the sap [balsam]). Tolu had a plasticlike consistency. The thick exudates contained ester resins, chiefly toluresionotannol cinnamate. Balsam of tolu was an ingredient in compound benzoin tincture.

Tolu and rock candy were added to rye whiskey to treat consumption, as an expectorant, as a flavoring, and for cough. As an inhalant, it was used to treat croup.

## TULIP TREE (1820–1882)

*Liriodendron tuplipifera*, family Mangoliaceae, was perhaps one of the most elegant trees in the American forest when in flower. The wood was compact, its yellowish roots, with the epidermis removed, were aromatic, pungent, and unpleasant to smell. The medicinal part of the tree was the bark of the trunk and root. Fresh root was intensely bitter and acrid and when chewed imparted a painful biting sensation almost like that of pepper. The camphorlike active ingredient, liridodendrin (terbinthinate), was extracted from the bark with alcohol and water. When included in tonics, it had stimulant, diuretic, and diaphoretic effects. It was used for intermittents, rheumatism, and stomach ailments, and worms; to abate hectic fever, diarrhea, and night sweats; and to treat—get this—hysteria. When used for hysteria, it was often combined with laudanum.

Tulip tree was officially recognized in U.S. pharmacopoeias only from 1820 to 1882. The powdered bark was dosed from twenty grains to two drams; an infusion was dosed at from one to two ounces. A saturated tincture was dosed orally at one fluid dram. Applied topically in balm form, it was used for cold sores. (78–alphabetical listing, "Tulip Tree")

## TURPENTINE (1753–1968)

Also known as purified turpentine (often referred to as rectified turpentine) and spirits or oil of turpentine, it comes from the pine tree, *Pinus palsustris*, and other trees of the family Pinaceae. Turpentine was prepared from oleoresin sap collected by cutting V-shaped grooves into pine tree trunks and attaching buckets below the cuts to collect the sap that oozed out. The process was the same as used in Vermont to collect maple syrup.

"Turpentining" took place in the late nineteenth and early twentieth centuries, with its peak occurring in 1915 in East Texas, where twenty-five turpentine camps existed throughout Jasper and Newton Counties.

A bled tree produced as much as a quart of the sticky resin per week. The buckets were collected and the product "stilled" like moonshine. Huge copper pots were filled with sap, mixed with water, heated, and passed through copper coils. The finished product was an oil that floated on the water collected in a tank below the coils.

Turpentine was used to treat puncture wounds—bullet, nail, plow cuts, and stabs from metals on which lockjaw spores proliferated. Lockjaw, or tetanus, got its name from the tonic muscle spasm and hyperreflexia resule in trimus (generalized muscle spasms), arching of the back, seizures, and respiratory paralysis. It was caused by the neurotoxin of anaerobically vegetating *Clostridium tetani*, with onset one or two weeks after the spores entered the body. Turpentine reportedly saved many lives from lockjaw. The accepted procedure for any metal cut was to soak the wound in turpentine oil.

The rectified form of turpentine was inhaled, or a few drops were taken orally (not recommended today) for chest congestion. It was taken on sugar, two to four drops, or in a tablespoonful of castor oil for pinworms in children. The rectified form was also used as a flavoring agent. It has been approved in the United States in extremely small amounts (0.002 percent) as a flavoring agent.

As little as a tablespoonful of unrectified oil can be lethal by causing pulmonary edema. Both forms were used in many topical liniments of old.

The hard residue left over from the distillation process was called rosin and had many nonmedical uses. Bull riders use it on their gloves to keep their grip. Fiddle players use it on their bows. The next time you hear a good version of "The Devil Went Down to Georgia," be cognizant that this old rosin was used in frontier times as a medicine.

Pure turpentine oil is still popular today as a paint thinner, but for all practical purposes, its use as a medicine has ceased. (4; 30–accessed August 13, 2002; 31–p. 83)

## UNICORN HORN (NO DATES—SORRY)

It is interesting to see how many times this fictitious ingredient was included in ancient medical treatments. Far be it to know what was actually given. Horny unicorns don't just roam everywhere. I found no record of their existence here in Texas, anyway. I did hear an account where a man swears he sighted one in the Big Bend area. The mescal he reportedly chewed may have helped. I'm told them little cactus buttons can make sight and other senses quite acute.

Extant to a letter written on March 21, 1595, powdered unicorn horn was used to treat Sir Unton, ambassador to Queen Elizabeth. The letter stated, "The king's physicians gave him confectio alcarmas compounded of musk, amber, gold, pearl, and unicorn's horn, with a pigeon applied to his side, and all other means that art could devise." Nonetheless, Unton died, probably from appendicitis or pneumonia.

## UREA

Ask any true southerner what the treatment for bull nettle sting is, and you'll get the same answer every time: "Wye, you pee on it."

That is the gospel. This old treatment has been passed down for centuries—in the South, anyway—from grandfather to grandchild.

Urine as a relief had many uses in frontier times. Aside from nettle stings, it was used in poultices with spit-wet snuff or chewing tobacco for wasp, spider, and other insect bites. Urine was a versatile liquid for the pioneer. It was poured (or aimed) down the barrels of muskets to dissolve black powder residues. It was also applied to animal hides to help cure them.

The chemical urea and other salty by-products found in raw urine inactivate the irritating toxins in the nettle's needles. Granted, it was a bit yucky to apply, but it did and still does work.

Today, urea as the carbamide is available as the active ingredient in numerous preparations used to treat nail destruction and dissolution and to remove dystrophic and potentially disabling finger- and toenails without local anesthesia or surgery. Urea promotes hydration, removes excess keratin in dry skin, and is very effective for other hyperkerototic conditions. Ever used Aquacare, Carmol 20, Nutraplus, or Ultra Mide 25 creams or lotions? If you have, you did what southerners have been doing to themselves for years. (1; 10)

## UVA URSI (1753 TO DATE)

Also known as bearberries, wild cranberries, and mountain cranberries, uva ursi berries were a favorite food of bears. The Latin word *uva* means "grape or berry"; *ursi* means "bear," as in *Ursi horibillis*, the scientific name for the grizzly bear. The berry was used to stimulate healthy urine flow and was thought to have antiseptic properties on the bladder. No records were available to prove or disprove these indications.

## VALERIAN (1753 TO DATE)

Valerian was and is the worst-smelling herb ever. It smells like the soggy socks of an old cowboy who has been three months on the trail without a bath. Much ado is made today over the placebo effect of some medicines. Valerian, *Valeriana officinalis*, family Valerianaceae, was one of those frontier placebos that had very little therapeutic value other than as a "one-doser" cure. One-doser cures were medicines that tasted so bad you got well, or at least said you did, just so you wouldn't have to take another dose. Its terrible odor comes from bornyl valerate and other glycoside constituents.

Valerian was used as a nervine to make you "rest" and for hysteria. Prepared in teas by steeping a half a teaspoonful in a mug of boiling water and straining, it was taken for excitability, migraine, and rheumatism. Anyone who has ever sipped Valerian tea knows full well that it'll gag a full-grown buzzard. It's hysterical, all right. Just watching someone try and drink it will put you on your knees. (4–p. 1052)

## WITCH HAZEL

*Hamamelis virginiana*, family Hamamelidaceae, was a small shrub that grew in Texas, particularly in low, damp woods. The leaves and bark were and still are collected, dried, and prepared in decoctions and infusions, which were used for their astringent and hemostatic (stops blood flow to the area) properties. Witch hazel was the old-time staple remedy and treatment for hemorrhoids. (1–p. 169)

## YUCCA

Taken orally, powdered yucca stalk was used by Native Americans for joint pain and scalp scale (dandruff). Applied in poultices, it was used on sores, to prevent bleeding, for sprains, and to help grow hair on a balding head. There are several varieties of yucca throughout the southwest: *Yucca schidigerea*, *Y. brevifolia*, *Y. mohavensis*, and others, of the families Liliaceae and Agavaceae. No active ingredients other than saponins (ingredients that have surface active properties or soaplike qualities, which make water foam) have ever been extracted from yucca. The Mojave (*mohavensis*) yucca was used not only as a food for Native Americans but as a foaming agent to wash hair with. (4–p. 1146)

## PARTING DOSES

Just as frontier medicines advanced with time, so did the laws. In the early twentieth century, the Pure Food and Drug Act of 1906 was passed. The law banned interstate commerce of mislabeled medications but fell short on quality and effectiveness. It took hundreds of deaths from the overuse of sulfanilamide finally to prompt the passage of the 1937 Food Drug and Cosmetic Act. Ironically, the act was actually too stringent and went so far as to include whiskey, hence the Prohibition days. Until then, medicines could declare to "cure" anything from falling arches to squeaky windmills.

The first patent application for a medication was filed in 1796 by Samuel Lee Jr. of Connecticut for his composition of bilious pills he marketed under the name "Lee's New London Bilious Pills" and "Lee's Windham Pills," which were sold throughout the United States. In 1804, Dr. Thomas Dycott set up a patent medicine practice in Philadelphia. He was famous for numerous concoctions and was one of the first to distribute medicines nationally. To keep pace with demand, he bought into a glass-making company. Today, collectors seek his intricately embossed bottles. Lydia Pinkham and her vegetable compounds aggressively advertised her remedies and began the "testimonial" era of frontier medical sales practices.

The word *cure* became a common household word in the nineteenth century. The federal government no longer allows the word to be used in medical advertising. And rightly so, considering the claims made by many proprietary medicine suppliers.

The manufacturers of the famous crazy crystals from Mineral Wells were ordered on Saturday, December 21, 1940, to cease and desist from representing their products as "cures." The Federal Trade Commission found that Texas wonder crystals had no curative therapeutic value other than as a laxative or possibly to help reduce stomach acidity.

But, as you see, many of the old lotions, potions, and elixirs did indeed have a sound basis for their use. And just as one recipe for apple pie is better than the other, how the old formulas were prepared had a lot to do with their success. Many of those old secrets died with the ones who prepared them. How you do it has a lot to do with the outcome. I, for one, have never been good at doing things the old way. I tried whispering to my horse once, but she just walked away. Obviously, there's more to it than just doing it.

It is a shame we have lost a lot of good remedies and how to make them. What with the political power of today's drug companies, many of the "good" old remedies will never make a comeback. There just aren't enough profit motives to promote their return. In defense of modern medicine, we are a lot better off today than our ancestors. Life isn't the lingering death it once was. Aside from its costs, the purgatory of the medical present isn't really all that unpleasant.

# FRONTIER MEDICAL DATES AND OTHER "WORTHY OF NOTE" FACTS

1747 Ben Franklin invents the "positive flow" theory of electricity. He also discovers that this "one fluid flow" can act at a distance.

1749 Abbé Jean-Antoine Nollet invents the two-fluid theory of electricity.

1762 John Montague invents the sandwich so he wouldn't have to get up from a gambling table to eat.

1765 The nation's first medical school established at the University of Pennsylvania.

1793 Alessandro Volta makes the first batteries.

1796 Samuel Lee Jr. applies for the first patent on a proprietary pill taken orally.

1800 William Nicholson and Anthony Carlisle discover that water may be separated into hydrogen and oxygen.

1802 First boric acid produced.

1803 Lewis and Clark begin expedition.

1806 Poet Elizabeth Barrett Browning born. Lewis and Clark begin return trip east.

1807 Henry Wadsworth Longfellow born.

1809 Edgar Allan Poe born.

1811 Harriet Beecher Stowe born; William Thackery born.

1812 Poet Robert Browning born; first recorded use of mouth-to-mouth resuscitation.

1813 U.S. Navy motto, "Don't give up the ship," uttered by mortally wounded commander James Lawrence of the U.S. frigate, the *Chesapeake.*

1816 David Brewster invents the kaleidoscope.

1817 Friedrich William Adam Serturner discovers the active ingredient, Morphium (morphine), in opium.

1820 Founder of modern nursing, Florence Nightingale, born.

1821 Faraday synthesizes tetrachloroethylene. Clara Barton, first president of the American Red Cross, born.

1822 Charles M. Graham patents false teeth.

1825 First appearance of homeopathy.

1827 First photographs produced on metal plate.

1828 Noah Webster publishes first dictionary.

1830 Paraffin discovered.

1831 Dr. Samuel Guthrie discovers chloroform.

1832 Hodgkin's disease, disorder of the lymph glands, first described.

1833 Thomas Davenport invents electric motor.

1834 Phenol (carbolic acid) discovered.

1835 Pepsin, the powerful ferment in gastric juice, recognized.

1837 Electric telegraph invented. First African American, James McCune Smith, earns medical degree from the University of Glasgow. Smallpox epidemic kills fifteen thousand Indians along Missouri River.

1838 Samuel Morse first demonstrates telegraph.

1839 First flexible stethoscope invented. First electric clock built. First bicycle constructed.

1841 First president to die in office, William Henry Harrison, dies of pneumonia one month after being sworn in. Oliver Wendell Holmes born.

1842 Ether first used as anesthetic by Dr. Crawford Williamson Long in Jefferson, Georgia.

1843 Yellow fever kills thirteen thousand in Mississippi Valley.

1844 Nitrous oxide (laughing gas) first demonstrated.

1845 Quinine isolated from plants.

1846 William T. Morton, D.D.S., performs jaw surgery using ether as anesthetic.

1847 First woman, Elizabeth Blackwell, accepted to a U.S. medical school. American Medical Association founded.

1849 Edgar Allan Poe dies.

1850 Nathaniel Hawthorne publishes *The Scarlet Letter.*

1852 Harriet Beecher Stowe publishes *Uncle Tom's Cabin.*

1853 Hypodermic needle first used for injections.

1855 Binaural (using two ears) stethoscope invented.

1856 George Bernard Shaw born.

1857 Louis Pasteur develops germ theory of disease and proves fermentation caused by living organisms.

1859 The silver deposit the Comstock Lode in Six Mile Canyon, Nevada, first laid claim to by a prospector.

1860 The Marey sphygmograph invented (first clinically useful instrument to measure a patient's pulse). First dime novel, *Malaeska: The Indian Wife of the White Hunter*, published.

1862 Slavery outlawed in all U.S. Territories.

1863 First commercial internal reed duck call marketed by Fred Allen of Monmouth, Illinois.

1864 First African American woman, Rebecca Lee Crumpler, earns medical degree. Smokeless gunpowder invented.

1865 Carbolic acid demonstrated to disinfect wounds. Joseph Lister recommends antiseptic surgery techniques to control infection. William Butler Yeats born. Salvation Army founded.

1866 First female, Lucy B. Hobbs, graduates from dental school. First patent on a shotgun barrel choke filed by the Englishman William Pape.

1870 Selenium, cadmium, and lithium discovered.

1873 Gerhard Armauer Hansen proves leprosy caused by the bacilli *Mucobacterium leprae.*

1874 *Streptococci* and *staphylococci* discovered.

1875 Lydia Pinkham develops her vegetable compound.

1876 Alexander Graham Bell patents telephone. Wild Bill Hickok shot by Jack McCall. Jack London born.

1878 First gallbladder operation performed; James Francis Shober becomes first physician with a medical degree to practice in North Carolina.

1879 Listerine Antiseptic invented. Silver dollar becomes legal tender.

1880 First electric incandescent light invented by Thomas Edison. Helen Keller born.

1881 Billy the Kid shot and killed in Fort Sumner, New Mexico.

1882 Patent for first successful action pump shotgun filed by Christopher Spencer.

1883 Theobold Smith shows diseases can be transmitted by insects.

1884 First dissolvable pill developed by Dr. W. Upjohn. Hans Gram, a Danish physician, using gentian violet as a component, develops the gram stain for identifying bacteria.

1885 Dr. William West Grant performs first successful appendectomy. Mark Twain publishes *Adventures of Huckleberry Finn*. Statue of Liberty arrives in New York from France. Louis Pasteur develops rabies vaccine.

1886 William Radam patents his "microbe killer."

1887 Svante Arrhenius deduces that electrolytes dissociate into positive and negative ions.

1888 Leprosy Mission's Purulia Hospital founded by Rev. Henry Uffmann.

1889 Insulin discovered as being produced by pancreas, and preventing diabetes.

1892 Almroth Edward Wright develops antityphoid immunization prepared from bacteria harbored by the patient. Sir James Dewar of England markets first vacuum flask (thermos bottle).

1893 Dr. Daniel Hale Williams in Chicago performs first successful heart operation. America experiences first polio epidemic.

1895 The National Medical Association founded for black physicians.

1896 X rays (discovered by Wilhelm Roentgen in 1894) are used for first time. First motion picture is shown in New York. National Association of Colored Women founded by Rebecca J. Cole, M.D.

1897 Aspirin first developed by Felix Hoffman. Joseph John Thomason first announces the existence of electrons.

1898 Adrenalin (epinephrine) isolated by John Abel. Marie and Pierre Curie separate two highly radioactive elements from pitchblende, polonium, and radium.

1899 Ernest Hemingway born.

1900 Blood transfusions made reliable by Karl Landsteiner. James Moses Browning patents first auto loading shotgun.

1905 Einstein develops theory of relativity.

1907 Machinist Ole Evinrude of Cambridge, Wisconsin, develops first gasoline-powered engine for small boats.

1915 French army develops first camoufleur (camouflage) uniforms for use on World War I battlefields.

1917 Dr. Louis T. Wright develops intradermal injection for smallpox vaccination.

1927 Dr. William Augustus Hinton develops test for diagnosing syphilis (precursor to the noted Hinton–Davis test).

1928 Penicillin discovered by Dr. Alexander Fleming.

1936 First medical textbook written by an African American to be published, *Syphilis and Its Treatment*, by Dr. William Augustus Hinton, M.D.

# OLD AND NEAR-FORGOTTEN MEDICAL TERMS

THROUGHOUT THIS BOOK you have heard words like *hydragogues*, *alteratives*, *galactagogues*, *epispastics*, and many more. The spell checker on this old computer went into drooling fits trying to decipher some of the words. And rightly so, for *Merriam-Webster's Collegiate Dictionary* no longer includes them. In most instances, explanations were included when the words were mentioned. But when a writer gets his head down, his fingers get an uncontrollable urge to purge. Accept my apology if some definitions were skipped in the text. So, for your absolute, guaranteed, toe-sucking pleasure, here are the definitions of many old and nearly forgotten words that like many wonderful things from the past have been blown away by the winds of time. And by the way, the term *drug* here means any medicinal, agent, or a product.

Abortifacient. A drug that causes abortion.

Alkalies. Drugs that neutralize acid; known to stimulate skin cells and soften epidermal layers.

Alteratives. Drugs that aid the nutritional processes or change metabolism.

Anhydrotics. Drugs that reduce perspiration by suppressing sweat glands.

Anodynes. Drugs that relieve pain.

Antagonists. Drugs that physiologically oppose one another in the body.

Anthelmintics. Drugs used to treat internal body parasites, worms in particular.

Antidotes. Drugs that, physically or chemically, remove, neutralize, or counteract the action of other drugs in the body; as in treatments for ingested poisons.

Antiperiodics. Drugs that modify bodily functions by arresting further development of disease.

Antiphlogistics. Drugs that reduce inflammation.

Antipruritic. An agent that relieves or prevents itching.

Antipyic. A remedy for puss formation.

Antipyretic. A substance that cools and allays pain, as in one that lowers fever.

Antipyrotic. A remedial for burns or catarrh of the stomach.

Antispasmodics. Drugs that relieve muscle spasms, usually in smooth muscle, as in the intestines, bronchial tubes, urethra, and bladder.

Antizymotics. Drugs that halt, suppress, or arrest fermentation, as in the stomach.

Aperient. A remedy that promotes excretion or emptying of the bowel; a laxative.

Aphrodisiac. *Aphrodisiac*, as you already know, is a Latin word that means a drug, agent, or product that when taken stimulates sexual appetite.

Astringents. Drugs that are applied topically, which cause muscular tissue to contract by irritation and check the flow of blood and other secretions by shrinking tissue.

Bezoars. The name of certain concretions (choleliths, enteroliths, microliths, uroliths, or fecaliths) found in the stomachs and intestines of some animals (especially ruminants). An antidotal remedy supposedly efficacious in preventing the effects of poisons by drawing them out.

Billiousness. A symptom composed of nausea, headache, and abdominal discomfort, which can be caused by constipation. Formerly attributed to excessive bile secretion.

Bitters. A liquor in which bitter herbs or roots are steeped; usually, a spiritus liquid possessing intoxicating properties as distinguished from beer or wine, which have undergone fermentation.

Blisters. Drugs that produce inflammation of the skin.

Boil. A circular-shaped skin inflammation characterized by a red, tender, puss-filled knot with a central, sometimes fibrous core. Also called a *furuncle.*

Brash. An eruption, or rash, a sudden attack of sickness, as in a water brash.

Cachet. Tiny wafers made from bread or flour dough, formed into a small, shallow cavity in which a drug was placed. Precursors to capsules.

Carminatives. Drugs that help relieve stomach discomfort and aid in the expelling of gas.

Catarrh. Inflammation of mucous membranes with a liquid discharge, more particularly of the throat and head.

Cathartics. Drugs that evacuate the bowel.

Cholagogue. An agent that stimulates the flow of bile.

Coccus. Also known as *cochineal.* Dried female insects that grow on cactus, the powdered bodies of which contain a red, water-soluble coloring. Often used by Native Americans in war paint, in artwork, or on festive decorations.

Comminute. To make smaller or finer, as in to reduce a substance like a drug by breaking, pounding, rasping, grinding, or pulverizing it into minute particles.

Concretion. The process by which soft or liquid elements become thick, solid, or rock hard; the act of growing together by a natural process; the formation of small particles of matter into a mass; a solidification, condensation, coagulation, or induration forming into a clot or lump of solid material.

Costive. Having difficult or infrequent evacuation of the bowels; *costiveness* refers to being constipated.

Counterirritants. Drugs that improve blood circulation, promote healing, and improve metabolism in the skin.

Decoct. The act of boiling a substance in water for the purpose of extracting its salient properties; to impart strength or warmth to a substance by boiling.

Demulcent. A soothing emollient.

Diachylon. A plaster, originally made up of plant juices, but later was made up of lead oxide and oil.

Diaphoretic. Drugs used to promote sweating.

Diuretic. Drugs used to increase urine flow.

Draught. A compound infusion of a drug; a steeping of a substance in water to obtain its active principles.

Dyspepsia. Indigestion caused by improper food digestion.

Elution or elutriation. The cold removal of soluble matter by washing with water, as in separating substances (foreign particles or impurities) by suspending them in the water by shaking, letting sit, then pouring off the water that contains the suspended particles.

Embrocation. A liquid medicine applied to the surface of the body; a liquid medication applied externally.

Emetics. Drugs used to induce vomiting.

Emollient. A warm, external application of an oleaginous, starchy, or mucilaginous nature, which allays irritation and alleviates soreness or swelling or pain.

Empyruematic. An agent having a burned smell; the odor of animal or plant substances when burned or subjected to distillation.

Emulsion. A soft liquid remedy of the color of milk prepared by mixing oil into water by means of a surfactant, which stabilizes the final product.

Enterolith. A concretion that forms in the intestines of mammals.

Eructation. To belch or eject wind from the stomach. Usually preceded or accompanied by pain or discomfort.

Excoriation. A superficial loss of skin by scratching or rubbing; self-induced skin lesions inflicted by physical means: as by the fingernails.

Expectorants. Drugs used to liquefy mucous secretions and loosen phlegm.

Fomentation. The act of applying warm liquors to a part of the body by means of flannels dipped in hot water with or without medicinal decoctions and wrung out. They were applied to the skin to ease pain.

Furuncle. A superficial swelling, usually puss and fiber filled, deep red, hard, circular, and tender to the touch. Also called a *boil.*

Gastrotonic. A drug that produces or restores the normal tone or action of the gastrointestinal system.

Gill. A liquid form of measurement; 1 gill equals approximately 8 tablespoonfuls, 120 milliliters, or 4 ounces (approximately one coffee cup full).

Granulation. The mechanical division of metals by stirring the melted metal until it cools while pouring it into a container rubbed with chalk then flaking the mass until it forms into rattling granules, which are then washed to remove the chalk.

Intermittents. A fever characterized by a more or less regular recurrence with periods of abatement, as in the fever of ague.

Konseal. A commercial form of cachets provided in kits to early physicians. A vehicle used to give medicine. Like cachets, they were moistened and/or chewed and swallowed with water. Intermediate forms of capsules.

Levigation. Trituration by the addition of water or wine to form a paste, which is rubbed until sufficiently smooth.

Macerate. To soften a solid by soaking until the constituent elements are soft and separate, as in steeping in a cold or hot liquid.

Madstones. *See* Bezoars.

Malactic. An emollient or softening agent used to soothe skin.

Nervine. A medicine that affects the nerves, as in an opiate, a narcotic, or a stimulant.

Obtundant. An agent having the power to dull sensibility or soothe tooth pain; a partially anesthetic medication.

Osseous. Boney; composed of bone; resembling bone.

Pectoral. A drug used to treat, cure, or relieve complaints pertaining to the lungs and breasts, as in an expectorant.

Phail. A handheld electrical instrument used as a medicine.

Philter. A drug potion, charm, or amulet that had the power to arouse sexual passion; a potion usually credited with magical or mystical power.

Pottage. A soup or porridge made by boiling herbs in water.

Purgatives. Drugs used to evacuate the gastrointestinal system via the bowels.

Purulent. Containing or consisting of pus or matter; involvement of the nature of pus.

Pyrosis. A burning, as in heartburn or gastric catarrh.

Pyrotic. A caustic remedy.

Rubefacient. A medication or agent that on external application produces redness of the skin.

Scrofula. A chronic disorder in which the lymphatic glands degenerate into ulcers, which heal with difficulty. It is usually hereditary though not considered contagious. Also called *struma* or *king's evil.*

Stomachic. A drug that promotes the functional activity of the stomach; a stomach tonic.

Sublimation. The process by which solids are, by the aid of heat, converted into vapor, which is again condensed in to the solid state by the application of cold; also, the act of directing the libido away from human objects to those of nonsexual nature—as in, "I got sublimated last night. She had a headache."

Surfactants. Agents that lower the surface tension of water, as in soaps used as laxatives and stool softeners.

Tetter. A once-popular name for eczematous skin diseases. Usually considered transmitted from animals to humans and characterized by intense itching.

Triturate. To grind by rubbing or bruising into finer particles, as in reducing a drug in particle size.

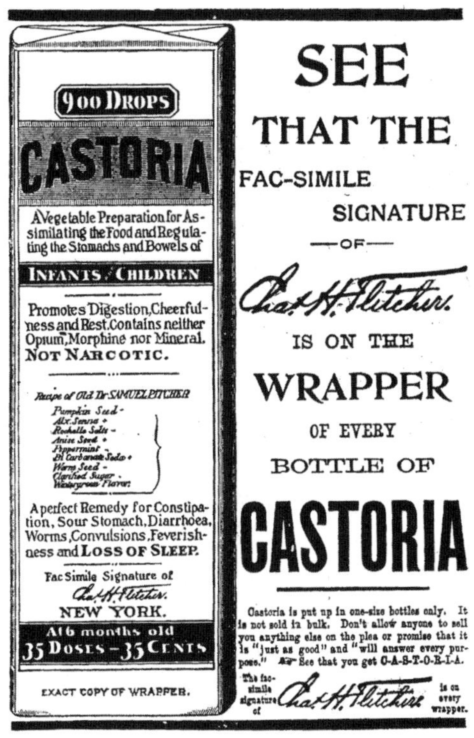


## CASTORIA

For Infants and Children.

The fac-simile signature of *Chas. H. Fletcher* is on every wrapper.

**Spoons Free to All.**

I read in the Christian Standard that Miss A. M. Fritz, Station A, St. Louis, Mo., would give an elegant plated hook spoon to any one sending her six 2 cent stamps. I sent for one and found it so useful that I showed it to my friends, and made $13 in two hours, taking orders for the spoon. The hook spoon is a household necessity. It cannot slip into the dish or cooking vessel, being held in the place by a hook on the back. The spoon is something housekeepers have needed every since spoons were first invented. Any one can get a sample spoon by sending six 2 cent stamps to Miss Fritz. This is a splendid way to make money around home. JENNETTE S. 13t

**The Laugh on the Sheriff.**

CARMI, Ill., Aug., 20.—A Kentucky sheriff got off the Louisville and Nashville train at this place this morning to have the manacles cut from his wrist. He had followed and captured a horse-thief in Missouri, and was returning with the prisoner handcuffed to his own wrist. While the officer was asleep the thief stole the key from his vest pocket and escaped, leaving the sheriff embarrassed.

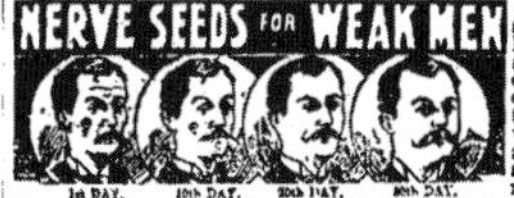


**This Famous Remedy** cures quickly, permanently all nervous diseases, Weak Memory, Loss of Brain Power, Headache, Wakefulness, **Lost Vitality**, nightly emissions, evil dreams, impotency and wasting diseases caused by **youthful errors or excesses.** Contains no opiates. **Is a nerve tonic and blood builder.** Makes the pale and puny strong and plump. Easily carried in vest pocket. $1 per box; 6 for $5. By mail prepaid with a written guarantee to cure or money refunded. Write us, free medical book, sealed plain wrapper, with testimonials and financial references. *No charge for consultations.* Beware of imitations. Sold by our agents, or address [illegible] Co., Masonic Temple Chicago.

SOLD IN BENTON KY. BY R. H. STARKS & W. [illegible] WILSON, DRUGGIST

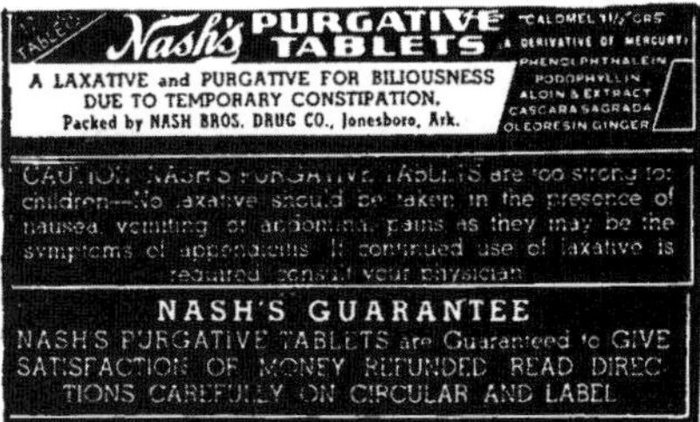

# RUINED!

Ruined by Rum! How many of your acquaintances? Aye, many. BROWN'S IRON BITTERS is the practical temperance medicine of the day. Not composed of liquor, not sold in bar-rooms, but a true tonic in every particular.

If BROWN'S IRON BITTERS is taken according to directions, it will not only relieve the intemperate man of the ailments resulting from his excesses, but it will remove all desire for artificial stimulants.

BROWN'S IRON BITTERS will cure Dyspepsia, Indigestion, Weakness, Malaria, decay in the liver, kidneys, and digestive organs. ☞ As a medicine for diseases peculiar to women, it is without an equal. Price $1.00. For sale by all druggists and dealers in medicine.

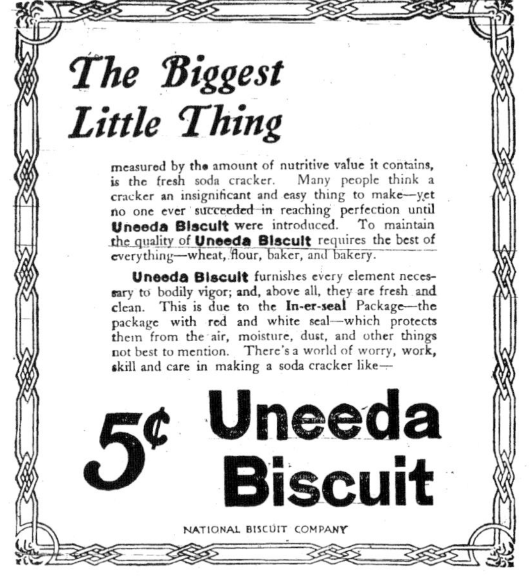
The Biggest Little Thing
measured by the amount of nutritive value it contains, is the fresh soda cracker. Many people think a cracker an insignificant and easy thing to make—yet no one ever succeeded in reaching perfection until Uneeda Biscuit were introduced. To maintain the quality of Uneeda Biscuit requires the best of everything—wheat, flour, baker, and bakery.
Uneeda Biscuit furnishes every element necessary to bodily vigor; and, above all, they are fresh and clean. This is due to the In-er-seal Package—the package with red and white seal—which protects them from the air, moisture, dust, and other things not best to mention. There's a world of worry, work, skill and care in making a soda cracker like—
5¢ Uneeda Biscuit
NATIONAL BISCUIT COMPANY

## SWEEDISH LEECHES,

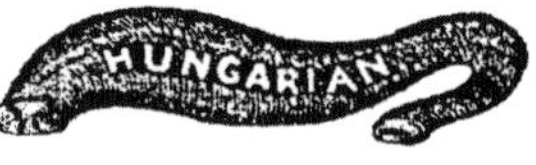


WE HAVE ON HAND, and Are constantly receiving fresh importations, of healthy Swedish and Hungarian Leeches, which we will sell at the lowest market price, wholesale and retail, at SYME'S Drug and Chemical Store, *91 Canal Street. N. Orleans*

## WEIGHTS AND MEASURES

### WEIGHTS, FOR DRY SUBSTANCES: APOTHECARIES' TROY WEIGHT.

| Pound ℔ | Ounces ℥ | | Drachms (Drams) ʒ | | Scruples ℈ | | Grains gr. |
|---|---|---|---|---|---|---|---|
| 1℔ equals | 12 ounces | or | 96 drams | or | 288 scruples | or | 5760 grains. |
| | 1℥ equals | | 8 drams | or | 24 scruples | or | 480 grains. |
| | | | 1ʒ equals | | 3 scruples | or | 60 grains. |
| | | | | | 1℈ equals | | 20 grains. |

### MEASURES FOR FLUID SUBSTANCES: APOTHECARIES' WINE MEASURE

| Gallon C. | Pints O. | | Fl. Ounces f℥ | | Fl. Drachms. fʒ | | Minims. M |
|---|---|---|---|---|---|---|---|
| 1 C. equals | 8 pints | or | 128 ounces | or | 1024 drams | or | 61440 minims. |
| | 1 O. equals | | 16 ounces | or | 128 drams | or | 7680 minims. |
| | | | 1 f℥ equals | | 8 drams | or | 480 minims. |
| | | | | | 1 fʒ equals | | 60 minims. |

The minim (meaning "small") is derived from the drop of water, which was once considered a very small dose; of watery fluids a minim is about a drop; of alcoholic fluids a minim is about two drops, and of chloroform and the ethers four drops are about a minim, as these are very much smaller drops.

### HOUSEHOLD MEASURES.

As the various spoons, wine and other glasses, tea and coffee cups, differ greatly in sizes, it is best when any of these are to be used for administering medicine to measure them with a graduating or measuring glass to make sure they are of standard size.

Household measures commonly used are given in the table following:

| | | | | |
|---|---|---|---|---|
| One teaspoonful | about | equals | one fluiddram or drachm | fʒj or 3 scruples. |
| " dessertspoonful | " | " | two fluiddrams | fʒij or 6 scruples. |
| " tablespoonful | " | " | four fluiddrams | fʒiv or ½ ounce. |
| " wineglassful | " | " | two fluidounces | f℥ij or ⅛ pint. |
| " teacupful | " | " | four fluidounces | f℥iv or ¼ pint. |
| " coffeecupful | " | " | six fluidounces | f℥vj or ½ pint. |
| " tumblerful | " | " | eight fluidounces | f℥viij or ⅔ pint. |

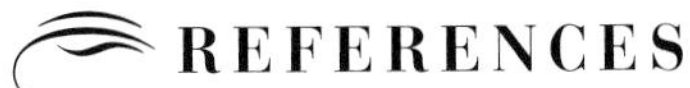

# REFERENCES

1. *Pharmacognosy*, Edward P. Claus. 4th ed. Lea & Febiger, Philadelphia, 1961.

2. *Pharmacopoeia of the United States*, 10th rev., 1920.

3. *The Herbal Pharmacy: The Interactive CD-ROM Guide to Medicinal Plants*, Brigitte Mars, Hale Software, 1997.

4. *Pharmacist's Letter/Prescriber's Letter: Natural Medicines Comprehensive Database*, J. M. Jellin, P. Gregory, F. Batz, K. Hutchens, et al. 3d ed. Therapeutic Research Faculty, Stockton, Calif., 2000.

5. *Materia Medica—Therapeutics and Pharmacy*, Kearney, Chiropody Record Publishing Co. 3d ed., 1948. Indexed Listings.

6. *Webster's New Twentieth Century Dictionary of the English Language, Unabridged*, Noah Webster. Publishers Guild, New York, 1950.

7. *Only One Man Died: The Medical Aspects of the Lewis and Clark Expedition*, Eldon G. Chuinard. Clark, Glendale, Calif., 1980.

8. *Devils, Drugs, and Doctors: The Story of the Science of Healing from Medicine-Man to Doctor*, Howard W. Haggard. Harper & Row, New York, 1929.

9. *Dorland's Illustrated Medical Dictionary*, 26th ed. Saunders, San Francisco, 1985.

10. *Facts and Comparisons*, Loose-leaf Drug Information Service, 1997.

11. *Early Folk Medical Practices in Tennessee*, E. G. Rogers. Nashville, Tenn., 1941.

12. *Dr. Chase's Last and Complete Work*, A. W. Chase. Dickerson, Detroit, 1895.

13. *Meriwether Lewis's Medicine Chests: Outfitting the Compleat Physician's Field Kit 1803*, Gary Lentz. We Proceeded On, May 2000.

14. *Blazing Trails to Wellness in the Old West and Beyond*, Gene Fowler. Ancient City Press, Box 5402, Santa Fe, N.M., 1997.

15. "Two Dozes of Barks and Opium: Lewis and Clark as Physicians," Ronald V. Loge. *The Pharos of Alpha Omega Alpha*, Summer 1996, vol. 59, no. 3, pp. 26–31.

16. "Illness at Three Forks: Captain William Clark and the First Recorded Case of Colorado Tick Fever," Ronald V. Loge. *Montana: The Magazine of Western History*, Summer 2000.

17. Texas On Line, www.tsha.utexas.edu; accessed July 25, 2002.

18. *Domestic Medical Practice: A Household Adviser in the Treatment of Diseases for Family Use*. Domestic Medical Society, Boston, 1926.

19. *Medicine's Great Journey: One Hundred Years of Healing*, Rick Smolan and Phillip Moffit. Little, Brown, Boston, 1992.

20. *One for a Man, Two or a Horse*, Gerald Carson. Doubleday, New York, 1961.

21. *Life on the King Ranch*, Frank Goodwyn. Crowell, New York, 1951.

22. *Talk of Texas*, Jack McGuire. Shoal Creek, Austin, Tex., 1973.

23. *Benton Tribune*, Benton, Ky., August 26, 1896.

24. *Diseases of the Skin and Blood and How to Cure Them*, 25th ed. Potter Drug & Chemical Corp., Boston, 1889.

25. *Colonial American Medicine*, Susan Terkel. Watts, Nashville, Tenn., 1993.

26. *The Medical Legacy of Moses Maimonides*, Fred Rosner. KTAV, Memphis, Tenn., 1998.

27. "Illness at Three Forks," Ronald V. Loge. *Montana: The Magazine of Western History*, Summer 2000.

28. *Ladies Home Journal*, January 1936.

29. *Meriwether Lewis's Medicine Chests: Outfitting the Compleat Physician's Field Kit 1803*, Gary Lentz. We Proceeded On, May 2000.

30. "Dairy Farm," W. T. Block. www.wtblock.com/wtblockjr/dairy.htm.

31. *Dr. Chase's Last and Complete Work*, A. W. Chase. Dickerson, Detroit, 1895.

32. "Traweek, Albert Carroll." *The Handbook of Texas Online*. www.tsha.utexas.edu/handbook/online/articles/view/TT/ftr30html.

33. "Seelye, Sarah Evelyn." *The Handbook of Texas Online*. www.tsha.utexas.edu/online/articles/view/SS/fse16.html.

34. The Vaults of Erowid. www.erowid.org/herbs/other/capsicum_info1html.

35. *The Indian Doctor's Dispensatory*, Cincinnati, 1812. See footnote 10 from reference 7 (p. 64).

36. *An American Doctor's Odyssey*, Victor Heiser. Norton, New York, 1936.

37. *Women and Medicine*, Beatrice Levin. Scarecrow, Metuchen, N.J., 1980.

38. *Women Doctors in America 1825–1920*, Ruth Abram. Norton, New York, 1985.

39. *American Indian and Lore*, Carolyn Neithammer. Macmillan, New York, 1974.

40. *The Doctor in History*, Howard Haggard. Yale University Press, Oxford, 1934.

41. www.applecidervinegarweightloss.com/history.html.

42. *Folk Medicine*, D. C. Jarvis. Crest-Fawcett, Greenwich, Conn., 1958.

43. *Woman Doctor of the West: Bethenia Owens-Adair*, Helen Markley Miller. Messner, New York, 1960.

44. Making and Using a Natural Dye. www.TexasIndians.com.

45. *The Kilmers of Binghampton*, John E. Golley. 1997. www.antique bottles.com/kilmer.html.

46. *Frozen in Time*, Nigel Bunce and Jim Hunt. The Science Corner, College of Physical Science, University of Guelph.http://helios.physics.uoguelph.ca/summer/scor/articles/scor243.htm.

47. "Gross Medicine," Maia Weinstock and Mark Bergman. *Scholastic Home Page*. http://teacher.scholastic.com.

48. CDC—Parasite Disease Information. http://cdc.gov.

49. *Infoplease Homepage*—"Encyclopedia"; www.infoplease.com. Hookworm, pinworm, tapeworm.

50. "Lincoln's Little Blue Pills." *Science Daily*. www.sciencedaily.com.

51. "Today in Science History." www.todayinsci.com.

52. "Peddling Snake Oil," Joe Nickell. Committee for the Scientific Investigation of Claims of the Paranormal. Investigative Files. www.csicop.org.

53. "The Saga of Jesse James," Linda Murray. *Hood County News*. http://granburytx.com.

54. "Perry Davis: Davis' Vegetable Pain Killer," Henry Brown. www.littlerhodybottleclub.com.

55. "History of Paracetamol." http://www.pharmweb.net.

56. "Herbal Remedies: Using Herbs Medicinally." www.liferesearchuniversal.com.

57. "Rio Tinto Borax: About Borax." www.borax.com.

58. "Early Southeast Texas 'Docs' Were Medical Men of Iron," W. T. Block. http://wtblock.com.

59. "Holistic Online Herb Information." www.holistic-online.com.

60. *Remington's Pharmaceutical Sciences.* Mack, Easton, Pa., 1980.

61. *The Edinburg New Dispensary*, William Lewis. Thomas & Andrews, Edinburgh, 1753.

62. "For the Female Discomforts," J. Ruth Dempsey. Helographic Inc. Transactions of the Royal Martian Geographical Society, *Journal of Historical Science Fiction Roleplaying*, Lydia Pinkham. www.heliograph.com/trmgs/trmgs4/Pinkham.shtml.

63. "Lydia Pinkham's Fabulous Compound." Good Old Days Online. www.goodolddaysonline.com/pages/stories/fabulous_compound.html.

64. "The Healing Tradition," Robert Gilmore. OzarksWatch. http://198.209.8.166/sheproom/periodicals/ozarkswatch/ow801c.htm.

65. "Rx from the Village Healer: Folk Remedies Gaining New Attention," Wendy Soderburg. *UCLA Today.* www.today.ucla.edu/html/900208folk.hmtl.

66. "A Modern Herbal: Anise," M. Grieve. www.Botanical.com.

67. *The Honest Herbal: A Sensible Guide to the Use of Herbs and Related Remedies*, Varro E. Tyler. 3d ed. Pharmaceutical Products Press, Haworth, New York, 1993.

68. *The Eclectic Physician Medicinal Herb Monographs.* www.eclecticphysician.com/herbs.

69. "The American Materia Medica, Therapeutics and Pharmacognosy," Finley Ellingwood. 1919. www.ibiblio.org/herbmed/eclectic/ellingwood/hydrargyrum.html.

70. "Nutrition." Aetna InteliHealth, April 22, 2002; www.intelihealth.com.

71. "A Modern Herbal," M. Grieve. www.Botanical.com.

72. "Calumba." *Clinical Abstracts.* www.Rain-Tree.com.

73. "Innovations/Copper in My Medicine Chest?" William H. Dresher. http://innovations.copper.org.

74. Traffic Dispatches Number 16. www.traffic.org/archives/march2001/musk.html.

75. "Eewahkee, Indian Medicine Clay." Educate-Yourself.org. http://educate-yourself.org/products/eewahkeedescrip.shtml.

76. "Specific Medication and Specific Medicines," John M. Scudder. 1870. www.ibilio.org/herbmed/eclectic/spec-med/plants-n.html.

77. "The Unusual History of Ether." www.anesthesia–nursing.com/ether.html.

78. *King's American Dispensatory*, Harvey Wickes Felter and John Uri Loyd. Ohio Valley, Cincinnatti, 1898. www.ibiblio.org/hermed/eclectic/Kings/quercus-lusi_nutgall.html.

79. "Gentian Violet." Healthyroads. http://healthyroads.com/mylibrary/data/altcaredes/htm/ame0230.asp.

80. "Japanese Honeysuckle." http://altnature.com/gallery/Japanese_Honeysuckle.htm.

81. "Prickly Ash." www.purplesage.org.uk/profiles/pricklyash.htm.

82. "Lye Soap the Old Fashioned Way." www.suncitysoap.com/oldsoap.html.

83. "Rattler Oil, Mesquite Beans and Prickly Pear." *Texas Electric Cooperatives, Inc.*, September 2001. www.texas-ec.org/tcp/901medicine.html.

# INDEX

# ABOUT THE AUTHOR

"Butch" Wayne Bethard (pronounced Beth'erd . . . he's an'erd, not an'ard, not a little Bathard or a little Bothered, either) is a pharmacist by trade, an author by design. He is by definition the truest of drugstore cowboys. He really is. He's a purebred, naturally inseminated, pedigreed, registered druggist, a hospital pharmacist, if you will. He graduated from the University of Texas way back when the diplomas simply said "The University of Texas," not "at Austin," or "Tyler," or "College Station."

Wayne is also a member of the Western Writers of America, the DFW Writer's Workshop, and a past member of the Texas Outdoor Writers Association. For three years he served as contributing editor for *The Texas Outdoors Journal* and authored his own monthly section titled "At Full Draw."

Wayne resides, practices, and writes out of his home in Longview, Texas, which he shares with his wife (going on forty years now), Wanda, a second-grade schoolteacher he still introduces as his "first" wife.